IT ALL BEGAN
IN A
GARDEN

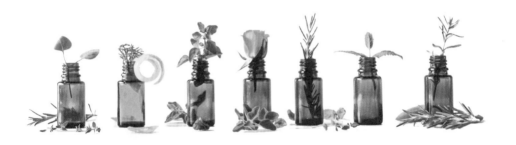

DAWN CAMP

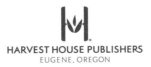

HARVEST HOUSE PUBLISHERS
EUGENE, OREGON

For those whose shelves are filled with and bodies are covered in oils,
for those who have purchased oils they don't know how to use, and for
those who aren't completely sure what an essential oil is:

This is for you.

Cover and interior design by Faceout Studio
Cover image of eucalyptus leaves © K.Decor / Shutterstock
Cover image of essential oils © by Dawn Camp
All other photography © by Dawn Camp

Readers are advised to consult with their physicians or other medical practitioner before implementing the suggestions that follow. This book is not intended to take the place of sound professional medical advice or to treat specific maladies. Neither the author nor the publisher assumes any liability for possible adverse consequences as a result of the information contained herein.

It All Began in a Garden
Copyright text and photos © 2020 by Dawn Camp
Published by Harvest House Publishers
Eugene, Oregon 97408
www.harvesthousepublishers.com

ISBN 978-0-7369-7958-0 (Hardcover)
ISBN 978-0-7369-7959-7 (eBook)

Library of Congress Cataloging-in-Publication Control Number: 2019054720

Printed in South Korea

20 21 22 23 24 25 26 27 28 / FCSK-FO / 10 9 8 7 6 5 4 3 2 1

ACKNOWLEDGMENTS

My family: Thank you for love and patience while writing this book.

Bryan: You make everything possible.

My local and online oils community: Every time you've said, "I need this book. Please finish it," you've encouraged me more than you know.

The novice oiler: I hope you find this book not only informative but also understandable and that it gives you the confidence to use your oils.

The skeptic: I've thought about you a lot. Keep your skepticism. Keep an open mind too. Oils are weird. As hard as I try to explain them, they are beyond words. Many of us grew up trusting the contents of the pharmacy, not the field, and it takes humility to admit there could be something to these little bottles. For Christians, it's quite an "aha!" moment to realize the molecules God gave us in the beginning—in the garden—work with our bodies better than manmade ones from a lab. God made them both: our bodies and the oils. He is not only the Great Physician, but He's the best pharmacist too.

Ruth Samsel: You've been with me almost from the moment the idea of this book entered my mind and you've championed the project ever since, like you always champion me.

My Lord and Savior, Jesus Christ: Thank You for this opportunity to point people to You and to the hidden gifts of Your creation.

CONTENTS

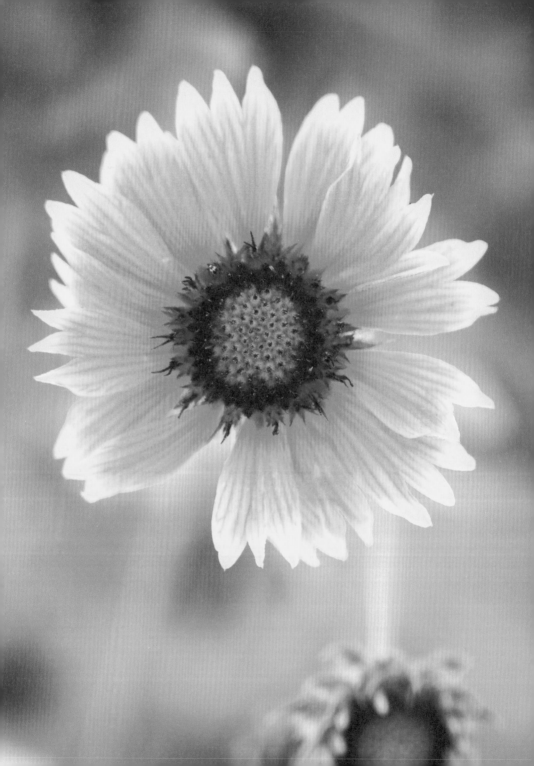

FOREWORD

by Edie Wadsworth, MD

It was 2013, six years since I'd left my medical practice to homeschool my kids and pursue my love of writing, and the first time in six years I was interested in reading something related to health. Maybe my medical school years cured me of wanting to study health and medicine, or maybe it had been so long since those kinds of books had inspired or given me hope.

In 2013 that changed. I began researching and could hardly believe what I discovered. A friend talked me into buying a box of essential oils. Because of skepticism, I mostly kept them hidden from my physician husband for a year. Surely there was nothing to the oils.

Interesting things happen when you're desperate. In the middle of full-fledged adrenal and thyroid crash, traditional medicine's answer (a pile of prescriptions) was not something I wanted at age 43. Oils and supplements, to my surprise, began to bring my body back into balance. Soon I felt better enough to hope, and I began making much-needed lifestyle changes. My body healed itself, and food and oils from God's garden were the catalyst.

Essential oils intrigued me. I spent the next year reading about and using them in my daily routine. The oils themselves were the best teachers, but I read books, journal articles, and medical studies. What

I uncovered mystified me. These were no snake oils, and they certainly weren't a fad. They were God's first medicine. Ancient cultures relied on them in daily life. They were carefully designed by an intelligent Creator to help with everything imaginable. And they were being studied in medical settings with astonishing results.

God made plants with healing properties. That's where most of the ideas for medicines come from. With the chemical revolution of the past 50 years, we have drifted away from simple, plant-based solutions to fancier, more complicated options. Thousands of chemicals fill the shelves of the processed food, cleaning supplies, and personal care aisles of your favorite big-box store. Most are made in labs not too different than those that make our prescription drugs. Interestingly enough, they seem, over time, to cause problems those drugs are meant to solve.

These chemicals are not easily recognized by our bodies, so we struggle to process them. Eventually, they can wreak havoc on our systems. When we stick with things God made, they tend to balance and harmonize better with the bodies He also made.

I'm thankful for modern medicine. Without a doubt, it has benefits. I'm glad to have an ER within 20 minutes of my house in case someone breaks a foot, experiences chest pain, or has trouble breathing. But if you drive down any main road in my tiny Southern town, almost *all* you see are pharmacies, doctor's offices, ancillary health services, therapist's offices, and more. Why are we so sick, and why is health care the number one growing business in the world? As a physician, I can honestly say we are pretty good at keeping people from dying but not very good at keeping them well and thriving.

We've gotten away from simple truths: Eat food God made, avoid most things He didn't, and when your body needs support, look for solutions that don't cause more harm than good (that may mean avoiding most prescription drugs) and ask yourself what you are doing in your own lifestyle to contribute to the problem. Much of what we face in modern "health-care" we bring on ourselves. Even most cancers are environmentally triggered. What we put on, in, and around our bodies is often the culprit, not genetics.

We have collectively and conveniently pawned our healthcare off to doctors, hospitals, and "professionals" in lieu of taking responsibility for what we do that may be causing disease. The new wave of interest in essential oils is a huge blessing to our culture, where we have become addicted to the Easy Button of processed foods and prescription drugs. Real food and real oils from real plants have tremendous healing potential for our bodies and minds. We are what we consume, either in or on our bodies. To move toward true health, look no further than the wisdom from God's first garden.

Adam and Eve were placed in a garden with everything they needed—most especially God Himself. We worship God, not His creation, but we stand in awe of the things He made and how perfectly they work in us to bring healing, balance, energy, and life. Essential oils renew my *awe* in God as a Creator and Father who cares for us in every little way. When I put two drops of frankincense in my palms, breathe deep, and let gratitude wash over me for these simple yet profound ways to support my busy, sometimes stressed-out body and life, I'm so glad I humbled myself enough to try them. I'm thankful for the person brave enough to share her "crazy" oils with her doctor friend. And I'm glad my friend Dawn listened to the call on her heart to write this book, which will comfort and guide many whose minds will be opened to this new and ancient way to support this one body and one life we have been given.

Because most of us don't have gardens anymore (which we would do well to remedy!), let's bring those gardens into our homes and enjoy the relief and healing they offer.

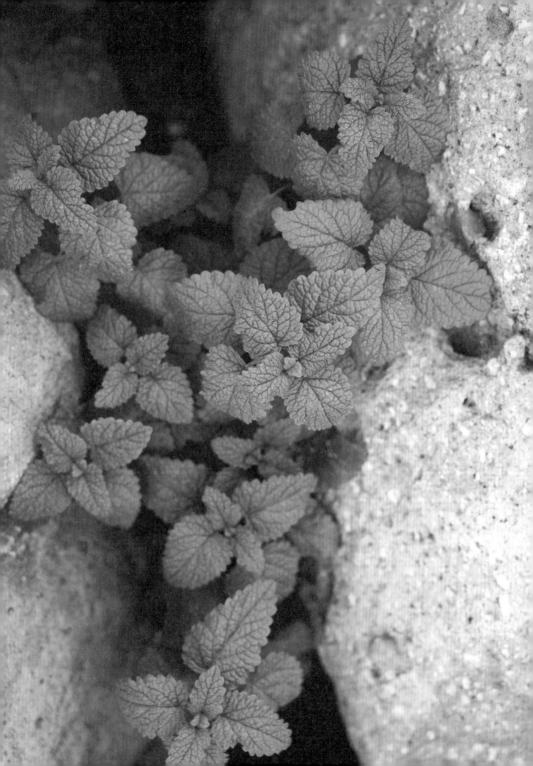

EVERYTHING WE NEED

There is treasure to be desired and oil in the dwelling of the wise.
Proverbs 21:20

Do you feel tired, stressed, and overwhelmed? In search of more peace, more joy? What if the solutions you seek aren't as big or hard as you imagine? What if health, hope, and healing could be found in something so simple that it fits in the palm of your hand? Second Peter 1:3 says, God has "given unto us all things that pertain unto life and godliness," including those things He introduced in the Garden of Eden. I've come to believe essential oils are part of those gifts, and by using them, we can experience less stress, more peace, and a greater sense of well-being.

Maybe you've heard the buzz about essential oils, but you're not entirely sure what they are. Someone offered you peppermint oil for a headache, a friend invited you to an oils class at her home, or a Google search recommended lavender oil for a sunburn. Or maybe you're a daily user of essential oils, and they are an integral part of your home, health, and beauty routines. No matter how familiar or unfamiliar you are with essential oils, this book is for you!

Essential oils may seem to be a recent fad, but they're anything but new. These oils are the most powerful parts of the plants from which they come, sometimes called the lifeblood of the plants. They contain natural chemicals that give the plant its "essence." When God placed Adam and Eve in the Garden of Eden, He surrounded them with what they needed to support their physical and emotional well-being through the essences of the plants, trees, herbs, shrubs, fruit, and flowers around them. Essential oils have gained renewed interest in recent years, but they are as old as the plants themselves. Ancient civilizations knew of their healing nature, and the Bible contains hundreds of references to essential oils and aromatic, oil-producing plants. Simply speaking, essential oils are medicines God gave us—a gift from above.

I turned to essential oils at a time in my life when I was stressed, my hormones were out of whack, I wasn't sleeping well, and I was dealing with unexplained pain. I had recently entered the world of book publishing. Two of our boys were about to get married. I was thrown into new roles and responsibilities as the mother-of-the-groom (times two), and my stress level was off the charts. The phrase "stress kills" popped into my head a lot, which wasn't a good sign.

One evening, at the end of another stressful day, I decided if there was *any* chance essential oils could help, then I was willing to give them a try. I'm so thankful I did! The combination of therapeutic-grade essential oils and a wonderful chiropractor changed my life.

Although I initially turned to essential oils for help with pain and stress, I discovered many additional uses, including:

* chemical-free alternatives for cleaning and for health and beauty products
* replacements for over-the-counter medicines
* potent and easy-to-store herbs and spices for cooking

- options for flavoring water

- ingredients in DIY gifts, such as bath salts and sugar scrubs

- help with calming a child

- perfume

- immune system boosters

- a natural air freshener in a diffuser

- sleep improvement and relaxation aid

- things to refresh my spirit

God is an intelligent designer. He not only created us but also provided these tools to help us live happier, healthier, and more abundant lives.

In the past, people spent more time outdoors and in contact with plants and the oils the plants produced. God provided them for our use and benefit. Why would He design us in such a way that we could only function properly with the assistance of man-made products and inventions? It just doesn't make sense.

Let this book be your guide on a quest to learn more about the capabilities of essential oils. Not only do they possess the power to positively affect the body, but they can also promote peace of mind, transform mood, or enable focus of thoughts and energy. As we explore each oil, I pray you'll see ways it can benefit you, whether you are an experienced user or discovering this world of possibilities. You will be amazed by the hidden benefits of the plants that surround us! May the stories in this book open your eyes to God's provision in new, exciting ways and always point you toward the Great Physician.

Blessings,

Dawn

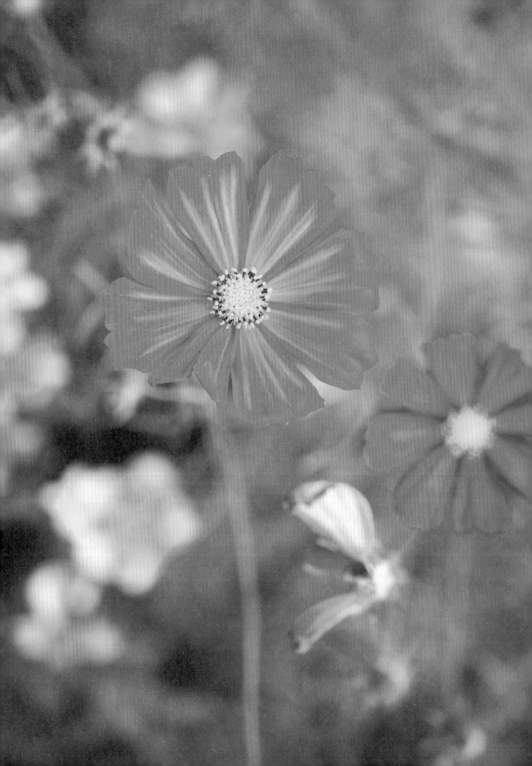

HOW TO USE
THIS BOOK

This book features 50 essential oils alongside encouraging, inspirational stories that correspond to each oil's historical usage, arranged alphabetically to examine in the order you desire. They were not chosen by accident but by their uses. It's a buffet of choices to help determine the oils you need to build your collection. In every offering you'll discover the wonder and wisdom of these 50 specific oils and learn practical ways to use them in everyday life. I'll share from my journey to encourage you on your own! Full color photos, diffuser blends, and DIY recipes for a variety of home, health, and beauty needs are also interspersed throughout the book.

What are Essential Oils and How Do They Work?

Essential oils are found within many shrubs, trees, roots, flowers, bushes, seeds, and plants. Extremely concentrated substances—60,000 rose blossoms provide only one ounce of rose oil—are much more potent than dried herbs and can perform within us the same important functions they provide for the plant, supporting our immune, digestive, reproductive, circulatory, and nervous systems.[1] When a plant is cut, the oils within it come to the rescue. Lavender is known as the Swiss Army knife of essential oils due to its versatile benefits to the human body. I'm an exceptionally bad gardener—nothing thrives in my care—so I was surprised to notice that the lavender I planted in my yard last summer looked fresh and healthy in the middle of the winter. The oil of hardy plants, able to survive harsh conditions, can impart its benefits to us too.

Essential oils are volatile, aromatic compounds comprised of hundreds of different chemicals. In this case "volatile" doesn't mean "liable to change quickly," like your toddler. Rather, it means "rapidly evaporating." Because their aroma spreads so quickly, I imagine them leaping into the air. My pastor once asked if I'd used an oil during the service. My husband had applied a eucalyptus blend to help his congestion, and apparently the aroma found its way to the pulpit. Because of the chemical structure and small molecular size of essential oils, they can cross cell membrane and move through our blood and tissues. When topically applied to the feet or soft tissue, essential oils can travel throughout the body in a matter of minutes.[2]

The exquisite fragrance of essential oils can help balance the emotions, lift the spirits, or create an atmosphere conducive to relaxation, focus, sleep, or romance. We run multiple cold-water oil diffusers in our home, and I wear diffuser jewelry most days. Before I refill a diffuser or apply an oil to my earrings, I think about what I will be doing that day or in that space. Do I need to hone in on a project that requires concentration? Am I preparing for a social or holiday gathering? Do I need to dispel odors from cooking (or smelly kids)? Am I trying to make our bedroom a setting for sleep or something else? Maybe I just want to smell nice or for my house to feel like a spa!

Essential Oils Safety

Some oils, such as peppermint and cinnamon bark, are called hot oils and may cause a burning sensation on the skin. (Other hot oils include basil, clove, lemongrass, oregano, thyme, and wintergreen.) Watch for redness of the skin in the application area, and always dilute the essential oil with a carrier oil— a fatty oil such as olive, coconut, grapeseed, sweet almond, jojoba, rosehip, or argan—when using for the first time, with children, or for those with sensitive skin. Essential oil molecules absorb rapidly because of their small size. Diluting with a carrier oil, which has much larger molecules, will decrease the possibility of skin sensitivity. You know what's amazing? Adding a carrier oil doesn't decrease the effectiveness of the essential oil; it merely slows its rate of absorption. Most applications require only a drop or two of oil—less is truly more.

Certain oils are photosensitive, which means you might experience skin irritation if you apply the oil and then expose the skin to the sun. For most undiluted oils you should wait 12 hours before sun exposure, but some require as many as 48 hours. Use photosensitive oils at night or cover the skin when you're outside. This group consists of mostly citrus oils, including bergamot, grapefruit, lemon, orange, lime, and tangerine.

Never use oils in your eyes or ears. If an essential oil gets in your eye, put a dab of a fatty carrier oil such as olive or grapeseed around the outside of the eyelid. Do not use water. Remember, oil and water don't mix. Water will spread the oil in your eye.

I would be negligent if I didn't specify that I only recommend pure, therapeutic-grade essential oils. Because the FDA has no regulatory definition or ratings system for essential oils, product labels can be misleading. A bottle can be labeled pure or therapeutic grade with only 5 percent actual essential oil content. We all love a bargain, but bargain oils are probably synthesized or diluted with a carrier oil. Consider it a red flag if a company sells all its oils for relatively the same price. You cannot produce a bottle of frankincense for the same cost as a bottle of lemon or lavender. Words such as "scented oil," "fragranced oil," or "perfume oil" may indicate a synthetic product. Pure essential oils are natural, plant-based substances. Synthetic oils are created in a laboratory. Be an educated consumer. Essential oils can replace chemicals in your home, so don't ingest or apply essential oils containing fertilizers, pesticides, synthetics, chemical solvents, or carrier oils.

I am not a medical professional, and the information contained in this book is not intended to diagnose, treat, cure, or prevent any disease. If you are under the care of a physician, consult him or her before diving in with essential oils. The information in this book is for educational purposes only and comes both from my research and my family's personal experience.

Please use your own judgment when deciding which essential oils to use.

OIL USAGE KEY

Aromatic

Topical

Internal

Hot
(dilute with a carrier oil; can irritate skin or mucous membranes)

Photosensitive
(do not use on exposed skin before spending time outdoors)

Avoid during pregnancy

Avoid for children under two

Avoid if you have epilepsy

THREE WAYS TO USE ESSENTIAL OILS

Three ways to use essential oils are: aromatic, topical, and internal. Each chapter begins with a reference key called "The Essentials," which shows the way(s) that particular oil can be used. Let's talk more about each one.

AROMATIC: Diffuse oil into the air with a cold-water diffuser, drip oil into your cupped palm and inhale, apply to diffuser jewelry (one of my favorites!), put a drop or two on a scarf, or inhale directly from the bottle.

TOPICAL: Apply directly to skin, preferably diluted with a carrier oil (more about that below). Oils are often applied directly to an area of concern, but the bottoms of your feet make a great spot to apply oils that can cause skin irritation or don't smell good to you because the pores there are large and the skin is less sensitive than other areas of your body.

INTERNAL: Oils certified GRAS (Generally Regarded as Safe) for internal consumption can be taken internally but only when labeled as consumable or as a dietary supplement. These oils can be used sublingually, meaning they are dripped under your tongue, or in empty vegetable capsules, which allow you to add your own essential oils. Essential oils considered safe by the FDA can be found here: *https:// www.accessdata.fda.gov/scripts/cdrh/cfdocs/cfcfr/CFRSearch .cfm?fr=182.20.*

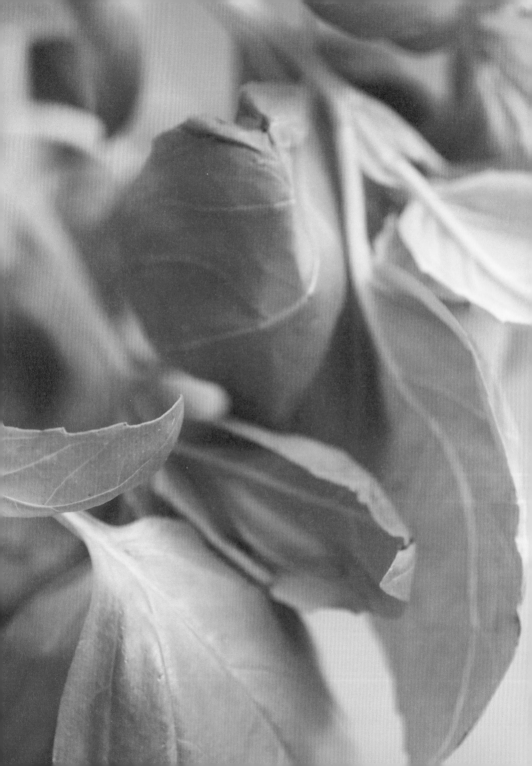

1

BASIL

The Essentials: *aromatic, topical, internal, hot; avoid during pregnancy*

If you thought basil was only a cooking herb, you might be surprised by the many practical uses of this popular oil. Essential oils are more potent than fresh herbs and more convenient to stock. For some recipes, you'll need very little: Simply swirl a toothpick in the oil to stir it into your recipe.

Wisdom from the Garden

Basil oil—steam distilled from the plant—makes a flavorful addition to pasta sauces, salads, or any recipe where you would use the herb. It has anti-oxidant and anti-inflammatory properties[1] and has been demonstrated to effectively inhibit common forms of multidrug-resistant bacteria.[2] Basil can increase mental alertness[3] and is commonly diffused for that purpose and is included in roll-ons for focus. Basil supports your respiratory and immune systems, soothes insect bites, relieves head tension, and can be combined with a carrier oil to create a muscle massage. Nursing mothers swear by basil for increasing milk supply (dilute and rub topically on the breast, away from the nipple, or take internally); however, it should be avoided during pregnancy. Basil can be used in the treatment of acne.[4] For menopausal women, it can increase estrogen levels and relieve hot flashes when mixed with a carrier oil and applied to the bottom of the feet or the back of the neck.[5] Basil is a hot oil that can irritate sensitive skin, so dilute well for topical application.

The fresh, herbaceous aroma of basil blends well with bergamot, geranium, lavender, or lemongrass in a diffuser.

Refreshment for Body and Spirit

Sometimes I imagine what it would be like to trade places with one of my great-grandmothers. I've raised eight children with modern conveniences: dishwasher, washing machine, air-conditioning, and a progression of vans from mini to maxi and now down to an SUV. My mother's two great-grandmothers each mothered a brood of nine without the perks that technology affords me, but they did so in what seems at first glance to be a simpler time. Common sense tells me they lived with different pressures, but pressures just the same. I've never depended on the work of my family's and my hands to feed us or gone without access to a modern grocery store. My great-great-grandmothers didn't raise children under constant vigilance to protect them from online predators and stresses. I've never delivered a baby into a world where infant mortality was common and without access to modern medicine. They never stayed up well into the night, under a deadline, eyes and fingers glued to a computer, seeking words to encourage readers they may never meet.

Ecclesiastes 1:9 tells us "there is no new thing under the sun." Moments, days, weeks, months, and years may pass, the physical and social landscape may change, but the form and function of our lives remain the same: food, home, faith, family, friends. We all need rest and soul refreshment, and even God Himself set an example of rest for us (even though He doesn't need it).

Basil oil lifts our spirits and refreshes us, provides clarity and focus, and soothes and energizes. It enlivens the food on our tables and relieves the fog in our brains. God knew we would need these rejuvenations in different times or seasons, and He faithfully provided at creation.

Infused Living

Add 4 drops basil, 3 drops rosemary, and 2 drops peppermint oils to your diffuser to create an atmosphere of focus and clarity during school time or while working on a project.

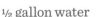

STRAWBERRY BASIL LEMON MINT WATER

½ gallon water

8 fresh strawberries

3 basil leaves

2 drops lemon

1 drop basil

1 large mint sprig

> Add 1 or 2 drops basil oil to spaghetti sauce for extra flavor.

Let water infuse for 4 to 6 hours prior to serving.

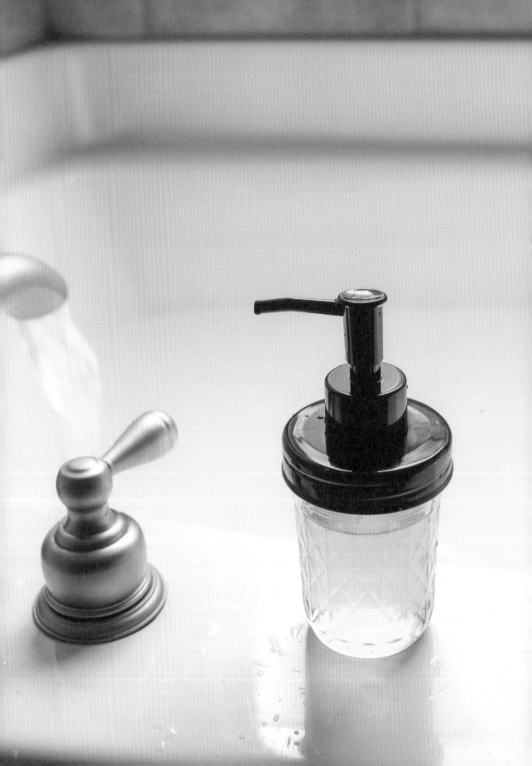

BERGAMOT

The Essentials: *topical, aromatic, internal, photosensitive*

Even if you've never heard of bergamot oil, you've probably experienced it in products including shampoo, perfume, skin care, and—my favorite—the distinct taste of Earl Grey tea!

Wisdom from the Garden

Bergamot oil, cold pressed from the bergamot orange, comes from a citrus tree grown primarily in Italy. The fruit is the size of an orange but looks more like a lime with its yellowish green color. Christopher Columbus is credited with bringing the tree from the Canary Islands to Italy and Spain. Bergamot essential oil is cold pressed from the peel of the fruit and has a sweet and relaxing fragrance. The components of this oil have been studied for their ability to relieve pain; to decrease heart rate and blood pressure; and to reduce stress, anxiety, and depression.[1]

You can use bergamot oil as a fresh-smelling deodorant option because of its antibacterial properties or add a drop to your moisturizer for oily skin, but remember that bergamot is photosensitive, so don't use it on skin that will be exposed to the sun for the next several hours because the skin will be more likely to burn.

The elegant aroma of bergamot blends well with lavender, orange, ylang ylang, jasmine, or geranium in a diffuser.

Guarding Your Stress Level

Recently I found my first gray hair. My first two, as a matter of fact. You can roll your eyes because this is not unusual for a 50-plus-year-old woman, but some of my family haven't had any gray until much older. It's genetic. Because these gray hairs were unexpected, I had to stop and ask myself: *How much stress is in my life, and how well do I handle it?*

When I fail to guard my stress level, two things usually happen: I go to pieces over small things or cry (a lot) during sad scenes in movies. (It's a sure sign I need a good cry when a movie triggers tears.) Left unchecked, high stress levels can affect sleep, weight, hormones, and even fertility.[2] Using essential oils is one of the best ways to cope with stress because they can lower the body's stress response. When we inhale essential oils, they affect our limbic system, the emotional part of the brain also connected to memory and our sense of smell. Bergamot is an essential oil known for its positive effects on mental health and well-being. Bergamot and similar oils help me dial my emotions down a notch and just breathe.

I begin most days with a hot cup of Earl Grey—my beverage happy place—and bergamot is the recognizable taste that distinguishes it from other teas. Adding bergamot oil to water or my diffuser during the day reconnects me with its scent and refreshes me in the same way. It may not keep gray hair away, but bergamot just might help you to cope with the stress in your day.

Infused Living

Create stress-reducing rituals incorporating bergamot oil and train your body to relax in response to its fragrance. Diffuse it in situations when you need to foster a relaxing and positive atmosphere.

BUBBLE BATH

½ cup Castile soap (if you use a coconut oil–free Castile soap, you may need to add some baking soda to produce more bubbles)
½ cup vegetable glycerin
2 T. water
8 drops bergamot
8 drops lavender
4 drops ylang ylang
4 drops geranium
8 oz. pump bottle

> Combine 2 drops bergamot, 2 drops peppermint, and 1 drop ylang ylang oils for an uplifting diffuser blend.

(Recipe courtesy of *recipeswithessentialoils.com*. Used by permission.)

SWEET CITRUS

4 drops bergamot
4 drops lime

HEAVEN SCENT

3 drops orange
2 drops bergamot
1 drop patchouli
1 drop rosemary

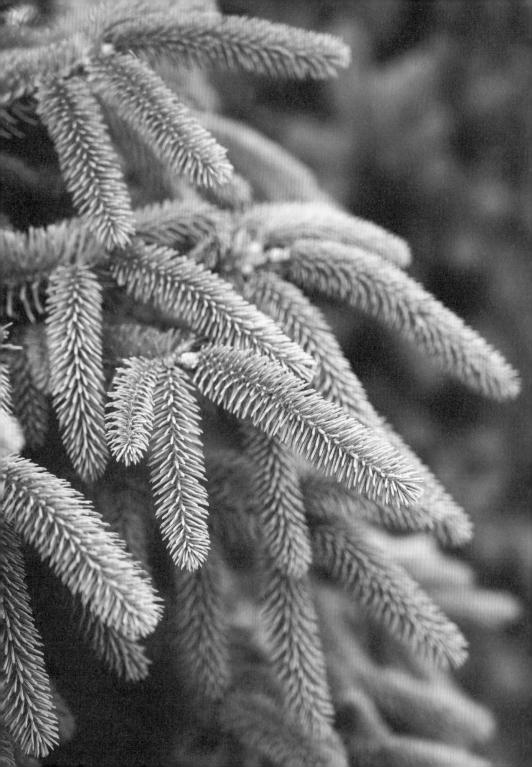

BLACK SPRUCE

The Essentials: *aromatic, topical*

The fabulous fragrance of black spruce smells like a year-round Christmas tree. If you, too, are a fan of woodsy aromas, you will love this oil!

Wisdom from the Garden

Black spruce oil, steam distilled from the leaves, needles, and twigs of the tree, has a lovely, grounding aroma that most find quite soothing. It strongly influences the emotions and can be used to bring about feelings of balance and positivity or help release emotional blocks. Add black spruce to your winter skin-care routine for dry skin and to enjoy its woodsy aroma. Black spruce can help with mental focus. Drip a drop of black spruce on top of your head—yes, really—when you need to get your head in the game. I love how its aroma lingers and emanates from my wrist (or the top of my head) for hours to come. Black spruce oil contains proven antimicrobial and antioxidant properties.[1]

Both men and women love the scent, making it a great option as a gift or in a perfume blend. Woodsy, invigorating black spruce blends well in the diffuser with eucalyptus, frankincense, and wintergreen, as well as floral or citrus oils.

The Blood-Brain Barrier

After using essential oils for a few years and experiencing some astonishing success stories, I've developed a great respect for medical professionals who consider them as options for their patients. If the objective is health and wellness with the fewest side effects, then finding safe, legal, cost-effective treatment should be the goal. Sometimes we fear what we can't explain or understand, but there are doctors and scientists who aren't afraid to explore the medicine God gave us, created to work in tune with the bodies He made. The internet is full of their research and discoveries, tapping into healing methods available since creation.

One of the most fascinating things I've studied in relation to essential oils is the blood-brain barrier, a filtering mechanism which protects the central nervous system (the brain and spinal cord) from dangerous substances and allows only extremely small molecules to cross. At one time it was thought to be impenetrable—literally, a barrier—but now the blood-brain barrier is known to be a highly selective membrane, more like a sieve. Essential oil molecules are extremely small and volatile. They leap into the air! Because they are steam distilled, only constituents small enough to be carried up with the steam become part of the essential oil itself.

This explains why someone can open a bottle of peppermint and a short time later you smell it across the room. Unlike synthetic drugs, whose molecules are too large, "essential oils of every species cross the blood-brain barrier,"[2] author David Stewart says.

Inhaling essential oils sends messages to the limbic part of the brain, which activates memory and emotions and our behavioral responses. Has an aroma ever immediately taken you back to a particular place and time or brought to mind a certain person? The scent of the lotion my mother wore when I was a child still brings warm memories of her to mind. The limbic system can only be reached through smell, which makes essential oils an extraordinary option for those with depression, anxiety, or panic attacks. Through our sense of smell, we can bypass parts of the brain that other senses simply cannot. Essential oils can have a dramatic and immediate impact on how we feel because they cross the blood-brain barrier and get into our bloodstream so quickly.[3]

The chemical composition and aroma of black spruce oil makes it particularly effective when you need to relax, focus, or balance your thoughts and emotions. It smells incredible. Don't underestimate the psychological and physiological impact of essential oils such as black spruce and their ability to positively affect your emotions.

Infused Living

Had a hard day? Combine a few drops of black spruce oil with Epsom salts for a relaxing bath or add it to a carrier oil for a warm, aromatic massage.

———

ATHLETE'S FOOT RELIEF SOAK

Add 4 to 5 drops black spruce oil to a warm foot bath. Its antifungal properties will help fight athlete's foot, and the soak can relieve pain and itching.

> Create a dreamy diffuser combo with black spruce, ylang ylang, and orange oils.

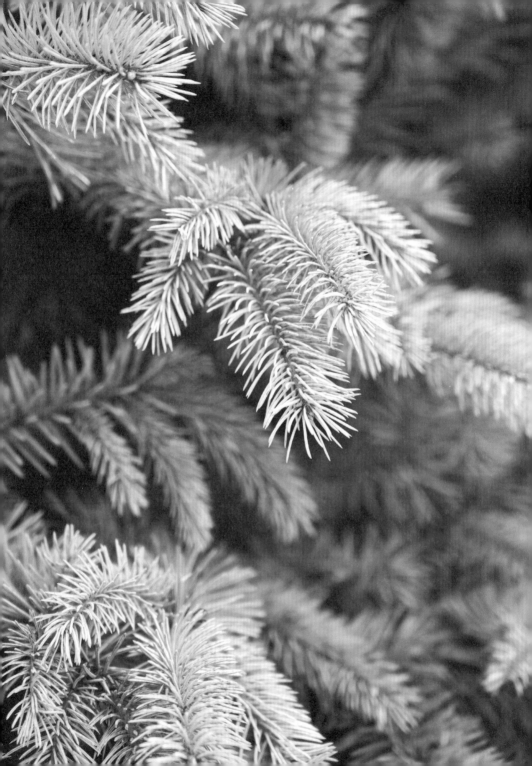

4

BLUE SPRUCE

The Essentials: *topical, aromatic, internal*

Blue spruce is a perfect introductory oil for men who want to dabble in aromatherapy. Its grounding and appealing scent boosts confidence and makes an excellent signature scent for either a man or woman when worn alone or paired with a fresh citrus or floral essential oil.

Wisdom from the Garden

Blue spruce oil comes from all parts of the tree—branches, needles, and twigs—and can rejuvenate both mind and body. It acts as a natural aphrodisiac, and when ingested can increase testosterone levels.[1] While we associate testosterone with men, it's important for women to maintain healthy levels of this hormone too. Blue spruce oil can provide natural pain relief. Native Americans used blue spruce trees for a variety of purposes, such as salves for treating wounds and skin conditions and as an inhalant for respiratory troubles.

The woodsy and refreshing scent of blue spruce blends well with frankincense, wintergreen, eucalyptus, or orange in the diffuser.

Confidence in a Bottle

I've often wondered if we fully transform during our progression from child to teen to adult, or do we simply become grown-up versions of our younger selves? The childhood me, who devoted hours to handwriting practice after receiving an *S-* (less than satisfactory) in penmanship in elementary school, sounds a lot like the adult me, who spent a day recording and rerecording videos for an online Essential Oils 101 class only to decide they weren't good enough and spent another full day recreating them all.

In many ways, as a child I was fearless: physically aggressive in sports, laser-focused on academic goals, and purposeful in my college search. When I set a goal, very little got in my way. But I became more fearful as an adult, and as a parent more aware of my faults and my failures, more aware of my depravity. I hate to be afraid, but sometimes I am. That's why one of my life verses, 2 Timothy 1:7, is so important to me.

My head knows the truth of this verse and what it reveals about the character and nature of God. When I acknowledge that the spirit of fear within me doesn't come from Him, it helps me to be brave whether it's in one-on-one friendships, a larger community, or any other area of my life. And when I shift the focus from whether I succeed or fail to whether I glorify Him or not...well, that changes everything. I love the story of two young Americans who won a silver medal for the United States in the 2016 Summer Olympics and then told the television audience that their inner peace resulted from knowing their identity was in Christ instead of in the results of the competition.[2] Let our confidence be in Him instead of ourselves!

Thankfully God blessed us with blue spruce: a dose of confidence in a bottle. Our modern lives are lived inside more than ever, but I can only imagine how the aroma of the blue spruce tree has grounded and emboldened men and women throughout the ages. My husband uses a blue spruce–based blend as cologne that he calls his secret weapon. Knowing how much it appeals to me increases his confidence that much more. Find out what this powerful plant can do for you!

Infused Living

Add a few drops blue spruce oil alone or with a complementary essential oil to a 10-ml roller bottle and top with a carrier oil such as coconut or grapeseed to make a special perfume blend for courage.

MOUNTAIN MAN COLOGNE BLEND

8 drops blue spruce
8 drops basil
4 drops Roman chamomile

Add oils to a 10-ml glass roller top or spray bottle and top with 80 proof vodka. Shake gently to combine before use. Use often. Smell awesome. Enjoy!

Add blue spruce oil to an Epsom salt bath or massage oil for post-workout relief.

WALK IN THE WOODS

3 drops pine
2 drops blue spruce
2 drops cedarwood

LOVE POTION NO. 9

3 drops blue spruce
3 drops ylang ylang
3 drops orange

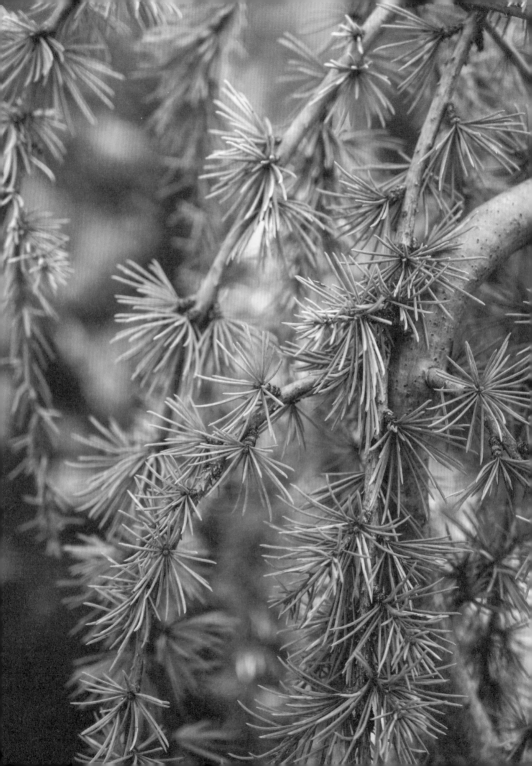

5

CEDARWOOD

The Essentials: *aromatic, topical*

Looking for ways to build your oils collection on a budget? Cedarwood is not only versatile—good for skin, sleep, and hair—but also economical.

Wisdom from the Garden

The Bible refers to both cedar trees and the oil they produce. Cedarwood essential oil, distilled from the wood of the cedar tree, can increase hair growth and combat hair loss by improving blood circulation to the scalp[1]—and it works beneath the scalp too! This woodsy scented essential oil stimulates melatonin production in the brain and can help ensure a good night's sleep.

The cedarwood oil contained in the wood of the tree repels insects, which is why it is used to make chests and drawers. In Psalm 104:16, King David calls cedars "the trees of the LORD...which he hath planted." King Solomon asked for wisdom and knowledge to lead God's people. He built the temple and palace of cedar, surrounding himself with the aroma of cedarwood, an oil known for its ability to bring focus and clarity.

He built the house, and finished it; and covered the house
with beams and boards of cedar.

1 Kings 6:9

Because of cedarwood's remarkable ability to calm the body while rejuvenating the mind, it has been used for children with autism and ADHD. [2]
Cedarwood cleanses and moisturizes skin and may be beneficial in the treatment of acne.

The fresh, earthy aroma of cedarwood blends well with bergamot, clary sage, cypress, eucalyptus, juniper, rosemary, and tea tree, as well as floral oils in the diffuser.

Emotion, Memory, and the Limbic System

As mentioned before, our brain works in fascinating ways, including the ability to connect scent with memory. For many of us, the combination of cinnamon bark, clove, and orange brings thoughts of Christmas. Catch a whiff of coconut and pineapple, and you can almost feel the sun on your skin as you recall the calm of an afternoon at the pool or on the beach. Scents can remind us of a specific person, place, and thing, or even a period of time.

Just as your brain builds scent connections, with time you can also train it to replace or build new associations. Take cedarwood, for example. If you've ever used a cedarwood-based kitty litter or hamster bedding, your brain may connect the smells associated with a litter box or hamster cage (ick!) with the smell of cedar. Cedarwood is used for its ability to reduce odors, but your brain may connect the good scent with the (associated) bad ones.

We diffuse cedarwood in our bedroom to help us sleep at night, but it's taken time to disassociate its smell from the pet cages my kids used to have in their rooms. One way I've done this is to blend it with other oils—cedarwood mixed with orange or lavender makes a pleasing diffuser combination. Repeated exposure to an oil can help build new memory connections. You can also apply the oil low on your body, such as to the bottom of your feet, as you adjust to its smell.

Many people report a better night's sleep when they apply cedarwood to their big toe or to the bridge of their nose at bedtime. A lady in one of my oils groups said her husband lifted her son's curfew because of cedarwood. When the son got home at night, the door chime on their home alarm system awakened the father and he couldn't go back to sleep. Once the parents began to apply cedarwood oil to their big toes at bedtime, the chime no longer bothered them. They were frightened the first time they awoke in the morning and thought their son hadn't come home! Add cedarwood to your oil collection and let it change your life too.

Infused Living

Add cedarwood oil to your diffuser tonight for a good night's sleep.

——

CALM DAY BACK-TO-SCHOOL ROLL-ON ⚗

10 drops cedarwood
10 drops lavender
10 drops vetiver

Add oils to a 10-ml roller bottle and top with carrier oil. Roll on wrists, forearms, or the back of the neck for a calmer school day.

> Add a few drops cedarwood oil to your shampoo or conditioner for healthier-looking hair.

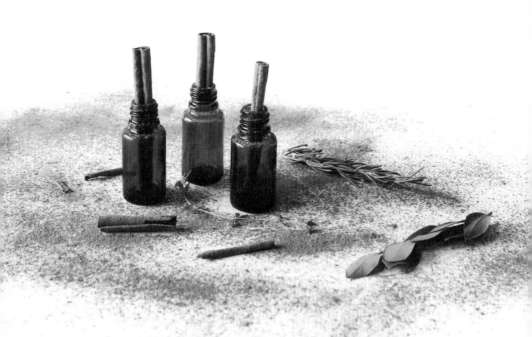

6

CINNAMON BARK

The Essentials: *aromatic, topical, internal, hot;*
avoid during pregnancy

Have you ever noticed how your brain connects aromas with places and feelings? Certain scents remind me of my mother, the beach, or my children as babies. Let the warm, sweet scent of cinnamon bark oil evoke fond memories of the Christmas season and comfort food!

Wisdom from the Garden

Cinnamon bark oil, which is distilled from the bark of the small evergreen tree *Cinnamomum verum,* native to Sri Lanka, is more potent than ground cinnamon. Less truly is more. Try a drop in your oatmeal for an extra spark of flavor. Cinnamon oil adds sweetness without added sugar, aids digestion, and boosts circulation.

Cinnamon oil can stop the growth of bacteria,[1] making it a wonderful addition both to household cleaners and to the diffuser to fight illness and support the immune system. Drink it combined with hot water and lemon oil for a sore throat, or diffuse it to dispel household odors.

Cinnamon oil has been shown to lower blood glucose levels and to be beneficial to insulin sensitivity.[2]

The spicy scent of cinnamon oil blends well with orange, frankincense, clove, tangerine, and nutmeg in the diffuser.

We All Need a Little Self-Care

My husband is selfless when it comes to caring for our family and rarely puts his needs before ours. If we need to cut corners, Bryan looks for ways to cut his own. It just isn't his instinct to put on his own oxygen mask first. He gets out of bed at the last possible moment on weekday mornings and showers at night. Breakfast is a grab-and-go affair—no time to sit! Morning and bedtime routines that require an extra minute or an extra thought rarely happen. I buy specific essential oils for my husband's type 2 diabetes, but many days those little amber bottles of goodness sit untouched. I realized the best thing I could do was to find a simple option.

I found a recipe that blends cinnamon bark, clove, rosemary, and thyme essential oils mixed with a carrier oil (I use grapeseed) in an empty 15-ml bottle, which I top with a rollerball, and wrap in fun washi tape. We leave it on his bathroom counter—where it won't be missed—and he rubs it on the bottoms of his feet and over his pancreas (just below the ribcage) first thing in the morning and last thing at night. Success! A simple self-care routine that works. Now he can take care of himself, and I can take care of him, because he takes such good care of me.

When Jesus says, "Love your neighbor as yourself" (Mark 12:31 NKJV), He implies that we look out for both. There's nothing wrong with practicing self-care. In order to take care of your people, you need to take care of yourself too.

Infused Living

Take time this week to care for yourself in a way that will also help you take care of others. Spend an afternoon curled up with a good book, make a coffee date with a friend, or schedule a doctor's appointment you've put off for too long. Dilute 1 drop cinnamon bark oil in 2 teaspoons honey and add to hot water for a spicy and soothing beverage.

CINNA-MINT LIP GLOSS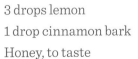

2 tsp. castor oil
¼ tsp. vegetable glycerin
2 drops cinnamon bark
2 drops peppermint

> Ditch toxic candles and diffuse cinnamon bark, orange, nutmeg, and ginger for a festive, fall-scented home.

Combine essential oils in a 10-ml glass roller bottle and then add castor oil and vegetable glycerin. Shake well for 2 minutes and then store for 24 hours to allow the oils to synergize. Shake well before each use. This luscious gloss treat is natural and chemical-free. Cinnamon bark and peppermint are hot oils, so expect a tingle. (The flavors will not fully develop until the gloss sits for a day.) Use within one year.

CINNAMON LEMON SOOTHING THROAT TEA

3 drops lemon
1 drop cinnamon bark
Honey, to taste

Add oils and honey to hot water to make a throat-soothing and immune-boosting drink.

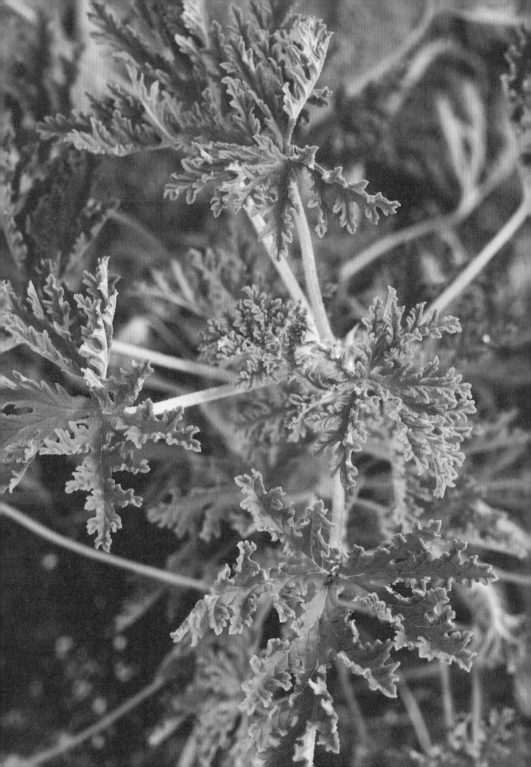

7

CITRONELLA

The Essentials: *aromatic, topical, internal*

You've probably heard of or used citronella candles, but did you know many contain as little as 5 percent citronella? Instead, use fresh, versatile citronella essential oil. It keeps pests away and so much more!

Wisdom from the Garden

Lemony citronella, steam distilled from the leafy parts of the citronella plant, is a natural for cleaning and disinfecting thanks to its antibacterial and antifungal[1] properties. Citronella not only repels mosquitoes around you but can also be used as a natural perfume, as an alternative to deodorant, and as a skin-care ingredient because of its ability to fight free radicals.

The fresh, lemony smell of citronella blends well with geranium, orange, lime, lavender, cedarwood, or pine in the diffuser.

Where I Talk About Detoxing My Armpits

I questioned the content for this chapter because it sounds a little weird and, to be honest, I don't want you to think I'm crazy. Detoxing my underarms has been one of my most fascinating experiences with essential oils, and it would be a disservice to you, my reader, if I didn't talk about it. Since essential oils entered our home in 2015, I've removed so many toxin-filled products and replaced them with chemical-free, essential oil–infused alternatives—shampoo, conditioner, laundry and dish soap, toothpaste, mouthwash, makeup, cleaning products—but although I started purchasing better options for the rest of my family, my old deodorant was one of the last health and beauty items I ditched. I couldn't find a natural option that didn't contain coconut oil, and I have a topical sensitivity to it. Going deodorant-free didn't seem like a good alternative for a woman in full-blown menopause, but it became harder to ignore the dangers associated with the products I used.

When my oldest daughter sent me a video of a woman using toothpaste as deodorant, I knew it was time to think outside the box. I use a fluoride-free toothpaste that includes coconut oil (I don't smear it on my face, so it doesn't cause a problem), and the woman in the video used a coconut oil–free option of the same brand. (Wouldn't it be funny if I used the same product in my mouth and under my arms?) From the day I put aside regular deodorant, I haven't used it again. Occasionally my underarms feel tingly from the peppermint in the toothpaste. If the skin becomes irritated, I apply lotion or an essential oil-based salve or ointment. It's important to understand that the process of detoxing and switching to a natural deodorant may temporarily involve rashes, excessive sweating, and odor because years of bad deodorants can not only leave a sticky buildup under your arms but also a surplus of bad bacteria.[2]

Now the skin under my arms feels normal—healthier than it has in years—and smells better too. Some days I don't apply anything and, surprisingly, it's okay. Many commercial deodorants contain aluminum. Mine did. One possible side effect of using commercial deodorants—and there are several, so please perform a web search—is the potential as endocrine disruptors, which affects your body's hormonal balance and reproductive system.[3]

Instead of adding to your body's toxic load, citronella, with its extremely high ORAC (Oxygen Radical Absorbance Capacity) value, fights free radical damage. This is an essential oil you need in your life and on your body!

Infused Living

Add 20 drops citronella oil to 4 oz. distilled water in a spray bottle to create a natural deodorant. Because citronella kills bacteria, it doesn't just cover up odors—it helps prevent them.

—

DIY INSECT REPELLANT

6 drops citronella

1 drop rosemary

1 drop geranium

1 drop spearmint

1 drop thyme

1 drop clove

> Diffuse citronella essential oil outdoors for pest-free grilling on the patio.

Combine the oils in a 2-oz. glass spray bottle and fill the remaining two-thirds of the bottle with distilled water and one-third with witch hazel. Shake well before using and spray on your feet, legs, and arms to keep away the critters!

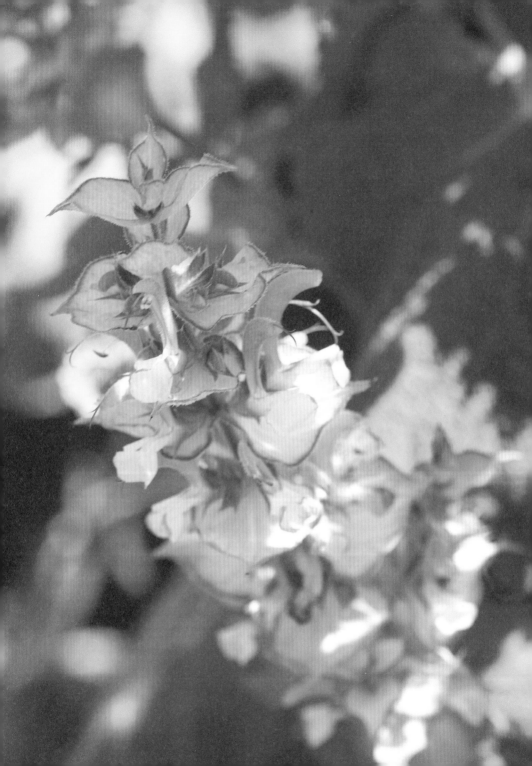

8

CLARY SAGE

The Essentials: *topical, aromatic, internal*

Ladies, our hormones fluctuate so much and affect us in so many ways, from the teen years through menopause. Thankfully clary sage can benefit us at multiple life stages. You need this oil in your arsenal!

Wisdom from the Garden

Clary sage oil is steam distilled from the flowering tops and leaves of the plant. In the same way chia seeds become slimy when wet, clary sage seeds have a mucilaginous coat, meaning they produce a viscous or gelatinous fluid when wet. This protects the seed from drying out, which would destroy it. Clary sage gets its name from the Latin word *clarus*, meaning "clear," because the Romans used this gluey fluid as an eyewash. A clary sage seed might also be placed in the eye so that a foreign object would adhere to it, making it easier to remove. (Do not try this at home!)

Clary sage is sometimes called the woman's oil because it can regulate women's menstrual cycles[1] and help with cramps, PMS, and supporting the circulatory system. It is a phytoestrogen, or plant-based estrogen, which is good, as opposed to xenoestrogens, which are derived in laboratories from petroleum and interfere with normal biological functions.[2] Clary sage creates a calm and relaxing environment, eases depression,[3] and may even stimulate creativity and help you dream. It helps to balance emotions and mood, and it can boost libido. Application of clary sage to the abdomen or inner thighs can relieve vaginal dryness.

Clary sage, with its herbaceous, grassy smell, blends well with bergamot, cedarwood, geranium, juniper, or citrus oils in the diffuser.

I Am Woman, Hear Me Roar

Although the lyrics didn't mean a lot to me as a five-year-old child when I heard them on the radio, over the years they have taken on a meaning for me other than what the songwriter intended. I've experienced the effects of hormones during my teen, childbearing, perimenopausal, and now menopausal years and watched how they affect my daughters and daughters-in-law too. I can say with certainty, yes, we women can and do roar.

Just like pregnancy hormones made me both sleepy and nauseated, caused my skin to radiate with that characteristic glow, helped with milk duct development, and caused the loosening of my ligaments and joints, hormones influence us physically and mentally during other life phases too. I try to remember that when my hormonal teenage daughters make me crazy. They may feel a little crazy themselves.

One day my daughter complained of pain in her lower abdomen. She had no explanation, but it hurt. I took one look at the area she indicated and had an idea what was happening. "Honey, you might be starting your period." Her response was a mix of horror and denial. As the mother of four daughters, I've seen some embrace this period (pun intended) and some not so much. This one dreaded it. She had plans to hang out with a friend that afternoon, and I knew the pain must have been intense when she lay down on the couch and said she wasn't sure she could go. A quick web search indicated clary sage might be effective for cramps—was it ever! Within a minute after its application, my daughter jumped up off the couch and said she felt better already. It has never failed to relieve her menstrual cramps.

My friend Melissa and I saw *Menopause the Musical* a few years ago before either of us had any practical experience on the subject. I thought menopause meant no longer having periods, but all they talked about was hot flashes! At the end, I looked at her and said, "I don't know about you, but I'm not doing that." Oh, sister. Little did I know that it wasn't my choice.

I knew with certainty that hormone replacement therapy was not an option for me. The risks are too great. I've found that when I rule out a course of action in advance, I work harder and more creatively to find alternatives. This has proven true in this area too. Do your research, and you will find that essential oils can help throughout the ages and stages of your life.

Infused Living

Put a few drops of clary sage on a towel soaked in hot water and use as an abdominal compress to relieve menstrual cramps.

___

CELEBRATION BODY SPRAY

2 drops clary sage
2 drops frankincense
2 drops orange
1 drop lemon
1 drop geranium

> Apply clary sage to the bottom of your feet at night to combat hot flashes.

Combine the oils in a 2-oz. glass spray bottle and top with distilled water. Shake to combine and before each use. Spray on after shower or when you want to feel fresh!

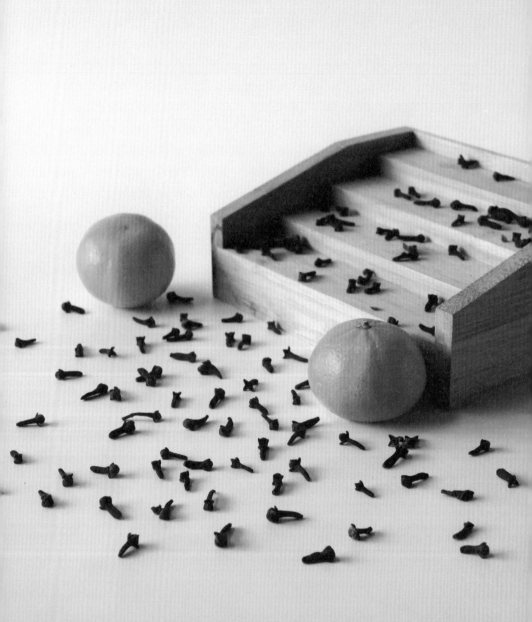

9

CLOVE

The Essentials: *aromatic, topical, internal, hot*

We associate the spicy, pungent taste and scent of clove with winter baking and beverages, but this sweet oil can do many things for our bodies too.

Wisdom from the Garden

Clove originally grew only on the famed spice islands off the coast of Indonesia, but plants were smuggled out in the eighteenth century, and today Zanzibar is the world's largest producer. The oil, steam distilled from the flower bud and stem of the plant, contains the powerful constituent eugenol, which is used in perfumes, flavorings, and medicine as a local antiseptic and anesthetic. Eugenol has known anti-inflammatory, cell-protecting, fever-reducing, antioxidant, antifungal, and analgesic properties.[1] Clove has long been used in dental care and can help prevent gum disease by killing two kinds of bacteria that contribute to it.[2] Clove (along with a balanced diet) may help balance blood sugar levels, promote bone health, and reduce stomach ulcers.[3]

The warm, inviting aroma of clove blends well with cinnamon bark, orange, nutmeg, or grapefruit in the diffuser.

Fight the Free Radicals

A few years ago the term *free radical* came into vogue. It popped up in phrases like *free radical damage* and *fight free radicals* and *the free radical theory of aging*. I soon realized it didn't represent a fringe political movement but was used mostly in connection with food and skin care. What are free radicals, anyway? In the body, oxygen splits into single atoms with unpaired electrons. Because electrons want to be in pairs, these singles—the free radicals—scavenge throughout the body, searching for other electrons to make them whole and stable again. The free radical steals an electron from part of another cell through a process called oxidation, which can leave its victim unable to function. Sometimes the cell dies. Sounds like an unhealthy relationship, right? Unfortunately, we're the ones that can become unhealthy because this process creates oxidative stress, which can weaken cells and tissues, and even damage DNA. It can lead to a range of diseases and premature aging of the skin, including wrinkles.

The body naturally produces some free radicals, but others derive from external sources, including exposure to toxic chemicals, air pollution, pesticides, smoking, and fried foods.

How do we fight back? Antioxidants, also known as *free radical scavengers*, can reduce the formation of free radicals or work to neutralize them. Without becoming free radicals themselves, they donate an electron to the free radical before it can steal one from another cell. A free radical, once stabilized, is no longer toxic to other cells. Hooray for antioxidants! Clearly we need them, which is where clove enters the scene.

Scientists at the National Institute on Aging (NIA) developed a method called an ORAC (Oxygen Radical Absorbance Capacity) value to measure the antioxidant activity of different foods. It's generally believed that foods with higher ORAC scores have greater antioxidant capacity, meaning they more effectively neutralize free radicals. Studies show that dried, ground clove has the highest antioxidant value of any herb or spice.[4] The USDA (United States Department of Agriculture), together with scientists at Boston's Tufts University, measured the antioxidant capacities of many foods, juices, and oils using ORAC values. Clove essential oil was found to be the most concentrated antioxidant with an ORAC value of more than 1,000,000. (In comparison, blueberries scored 2400 and oranges 750.[5])

While you may find disagreement about the importance of the ORAC scale, antioxidants obviously play an important role in protecting our cells and our health. My husband and I add clove to our nightly capsules because of its protective capabilities. God, knowing what our bodies need, provided for us through this common yet uncommonly extraordinary oil.

Infused Living

Put clove oil and a carrier oil on a cotton swab and apply topically to relieve a toothache. Watch where you touch, though, or you'll numb your lip or tongue too!

———

PUMPKIN SPICE CREAMER 🍶

2 cups almond milk

⅓ cup pumpkin puree

1 tsp. vanilla

1 drop clove

1 drop ginger

1 drop cinnamon bark

> Diffuse clove, cinnamon bark, orange, and nutmeg to summon the sweet scent of fall.

Combine ingredients in a blender until smooth. Store in an airtight container in the fridge. Shake before using and finish within seven days.

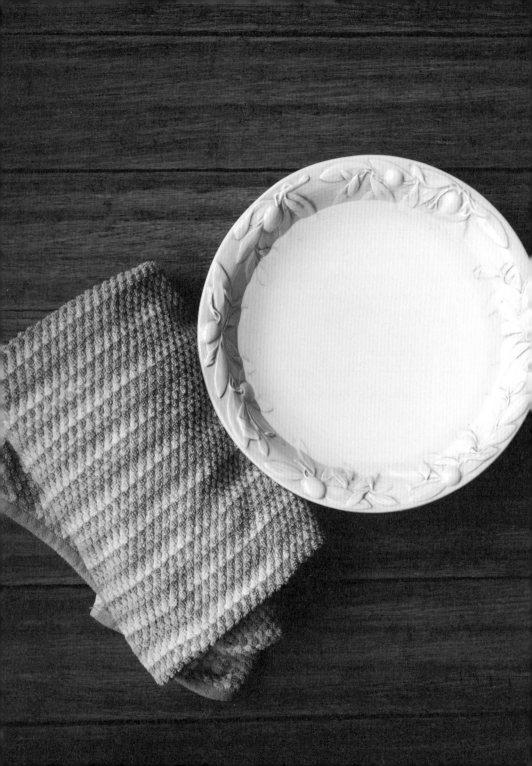

10

COPAIBA

The Essentials: *aromatic, topical, internal*

It took a while for me to learn how to use copaiba essential oil. Maybe because it isn't only for one specific thing. It works for almost everything! Besides being fun to say (I pronounce it kō-pī-ē′-bə), versatile copaiba amplifies the effect of other oils when combined.

Wisdom from the Garden

Copaiba has been used in folk medicine since the sixteenth century in its native South America. Steam distilled from the gum resin of a Brazilian tree, copaiba is a powerful oil yet gentle enough that mothers use it to soothe the gums of teething babies. Copaiba may be helpful for inflammation,[1] healing wounds,[2] reducing the appearance of acne,[3] congestion and respiratory issues, oral care,[4] and healthy skin when added to a moisturizer. Apply it to a specific location or add a couple drops of copaiba to herbal tea, warm water and honey, or a homemade essential oil veggie capsule for internal consumption. Copaiba can help calm you, clear your head, and focus your thoughts.

Combine the gentle, woodsy aroma of copaiba with citrus or floral oils for a custom perfume blend, either neat—meaning undiluted—or topped off with a carrier oil or vodka in a glass bottle with roller applicator.

Copaiba blends well with geranium, ylang ylang, lime, lavender, and cedarwood in the diffuser.

Amplified Effects

As a teen, the girls on my cheerleading squad teased me about my bowed legs. "Dawn, put your feet together," they'd call out as we gathered in formation to practice a new cheer. I'd reply, "They are," and then we'd all giggle. Before you decide my friends weren't nice, I'll tell you this was all in good fun. I have bowed legs, and so do my sons.

A few years ago when I needed to exercise more, I started running. I've never participated in a 5K or any organized event, but I jog in my neighborhood or on our county's greenway during my children's track and cross-country practices. Once, at the end of a fall morning run, I looked down and observed the way my feet strike the pavement at an odd angle because of the shape of my legs. Shouldn't they land in a way that distributes my weight more evenly? I consciously altered my stride to fit the model in my head, which resulted in months of pain in my right ankle. It was a not-so-subtle reminder to accept the unique way God created me instead of trying to conform to an imaginary ideal. During that time I applied a variety of oils that brought temporary relief but not a lasting cure. It was when I turned to copaiba, either alone or combined with other oils to amplify its effect (one of the oil's most amazing characteristics), that the pain finally went away.

Sometimes I place a drop or two of copaiba under my tongue to deal with stress or anxiety, or to wind down at bedtime. When you drip oil under your tongue, allow it to sit there for at least 30 seconds before you swish it around or swallow it with water. That area is capillary rich, and the oil will pass into your bloodstream faster than when traveling through your digestive tract. Copaiba is one of my favorite oils for relaxation or relief of inflammation.

Infused Living

If you're dealing with extra stress or pain, create a custom massage oil by adding copaiba to a carrier oil after exercise or a difficult day.

RELAXING FOOT SOAK

1 cup Epsom salt
2 drops copaiba
2 drops wintergreen
Warm water

Mix Epsom salt and the essential oils with warm water in a tub big enough for your feet. Relax and soak for 15 to 30 minutes.

> Rub copaiba (labeled for internal consumption) on a teething baby's gums for relief, with or without a carrier oil.

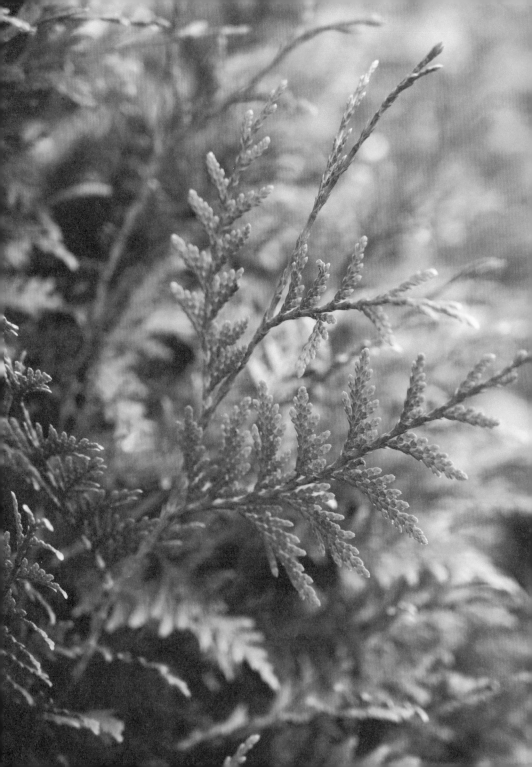

11

CYPRESS

The Essentials: *aromatic, topical, internal*

Woodsy cypress oil stimulates blood circulation. Mix it with a carrier oil (I use grapeseed) in a pump bottle to create a circulation-improving massage oil that can be used in place of lotion.

Wisdom from the Garden

The oil of the durable cypress tree exhibits significant antibacterial, anti-inflammatory, antifungal, and antioxidant properties and inhibits the growth of yeast.[1] It may benefit those with respiratory problems, and it contains camphene, a common ingredient in herbal cough suppressants. Because cypress is antibacterial, it can benefit skin conditions like acne and disinfect wounds, and because it's antiviral, it can fight warts. Cypress also has been shown to enhance liver and kidney function.[2] It improves circulation and may help reduce the appearance of cellulite. Blend cypress with a carrier oil and massage onto sore muscles[3] or rub on your lower abdomen (over your bladder) at bedtime to help sleep through the night without getting up to go to the bathroom or to help with bedwetting.

The clean, herbaceous scent of cypress imparts feelings of grounding and security and blends well with lavender, lemon, orange, juniper, or sandalwood in the diffuser.

Superstar Cypress

Essential oils are the plant's defense system, both in the way it protects itself from pests, predators, and disease and in the way it attracts pollinators.[4] Thankfully, essential oils impart benefits to us by supporting and regulating our body systems in the same way.[5] Many of the most powerful essential oils come from plants that live in harsh climates or are exceptionally hardy, like the cypress tree, whose botanical name means "live forever." According to legend, the doors of Noah's ark and the original doors of St. Peter's Basilica in Rome, which are said to have lasted more than 1,000 years, were both made from cypress wood.

When I think of cypress oil, I think of its ability to increase blood circulation by constricting blood vessels and tightening tissue. A friend who dealt with varicose veins and bruising during her pregnancy applied cypress topically to affected areas for symptom relief. Poor circulation is one cause of varicose veins, and cypress is commonly used as treatment. (I apply it to spider veins on my legs.) Cypress also comes highly recommended in the popular book *Lucy Libido Says…There's an Oil for THAT: A Girlfriend's Guide to Using Essential Oils Between the Sheets*, which includes many cypress-based DIY recipes. I vouch for the benefits of both the book and the oil. Along with its many practical applications, cypress also promotes feelings of grounding and security and can add an alluring component to an outdoorsy-smelling cologne blend.

Infused Living

Mix 1 drop cypress oil with 1 drop of the carrier oil of your choice and dab lightly under your eyes to reduce fine lines and puffiness. Be careful to never get essential oils in your eyes.

> Massage cypress and a carrier oil on your legs to increase blood circulation before running.

(Reminder: If you do get oil in your eyes, don't rinse it with water—oil and water don't mix, and water will spread the essential oil. Instead, try to flush the oil with a carrier oil or put a dab of carrier oil in the corner of your eye.)

___

ENERGIZING BODY OIL

10 drops cypress
10 drops grapefruit

Combine the essential oils and top with a carrier oil in a glass bottle with a pump. Cypress is good for circulation, and grapefruit helps get rid of the dimples we don't love on our arms and legs. Apply after showering the way you would use lotion.

SPRING DIFFUSER RECIPES

SUNNY-SIDE UP

2 drops tangerine

2 drops lemongrass

2 drops spearmint

WEDDING SEASON

4 drops juniper

4 drops lime

2 drops clary sage

SPRING FORWARD

6 drops grapefruit

2 drops peppermint

1 drop geranium

IN BLOOM

3 drops orange

2 drops ginger

2 drops ylang ylang

SPRING CLEANING

3 drops lime

3 drops lemon

2 drops lavender

2 drops rosemary

GARDEN PARTY

2 drops lime

2 drops peppermint

1 drop basil

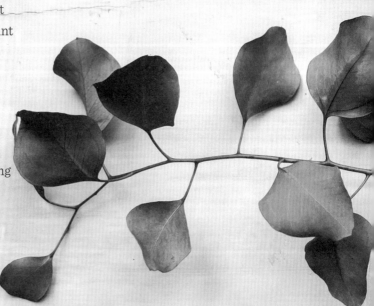

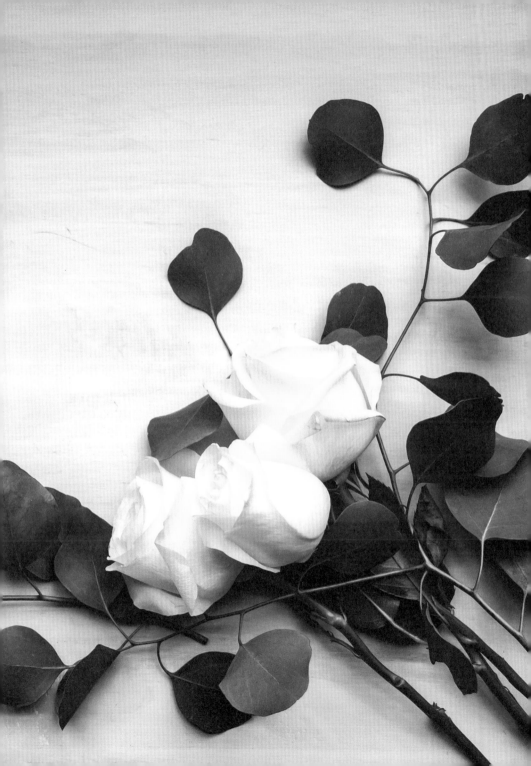

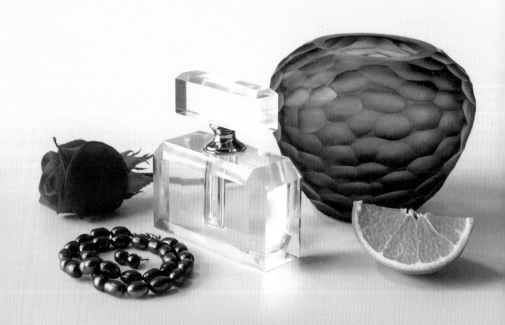

12

DAVANA

The Essentials: *topical, aromatic*

Want to create your own personal signature scent? Try davana as an interesting top note. Adaptive to the wearer, davana smells slightly different on everyone, so your fragrance blend will be unique to you.

Wisdom from the Garden

The davana herb, native to India, belongs to the daisy family. Its sweet, warm fragrance inspires a sense of comfort, calm, and contentment. Davana can help clear your skin and brighten your outlook. It's a desirable perfume ingredient because it adapts to the personal chemistry of the individual wearer. How davana smells in the bottle may be different than how it smells on you, and the scent may continue to change as it remains on your skin. Davanone, a constituent of davana, is being evaluated as a possible insect deterrent. (Smelling good to people but bad to bugs is a win-win!) Appealing, exotic davana is considered an aphrodisiac in some cultures.

The rich, fruity aroma of davana blends well with sandalwood, frankincense, ylang ylang, rose, geranium, or bergamot in the diffuser.

Know Better, Do Better

I remember the two perfumes I wore most in high school. My husband still recalls how I smelled when we met and while we dated. As an adult, I have favored a variety of popular fragrances at different times, usually wearing both the spray and the scented body lotion. Now I know that, unfortunately, these products often contain scant amounts, if any, of the natural scents they seek to mimic.

The aroma of commercial fragrances often comes from the combination of a dozen or more potentially dangerous synthetic chemicals, including petrochemicals, which are obtained by the refining or processing of petroleum or natural gas.[1] Does this sound as disgusting—not to mention dangerous—to you as it does to me? Please read this chapter carefully and do your own research. When we know better, we do better.

Companies in the United States are not required to disclose the ingredients they include in personal care products in order to protect their trade secrets. But who's protecting us? If these components were natural, it wouldn't be so bad. Instead, it gives manufacturers a free pass to hide ingredients from unsuspecting consumers who might be appalled to know they purchase for their families products that may cause allergies, disrupt hormones, decrease fertility, and more. Early exposure to phthalates, a chemical hidden under the fragrance category in a number of personal care products, can lead to lower thyroid function in girls and a host of other related problems.[2] Check your personal care products for known carcinogens and synthetic toxins such as parabens (including methylparaben, isopropylparaben, and propylparaben),[3] triclosan,[4] and talc,[5] and avoid any product that lists fragrance as an ingredient, because you can never really know what it contains.

It pains me to think of the products filled with synthetic chemicals I bought for my family for years, and that I put on my babies. I would love to say our home is now free of them, but it's hard to persuade people—even my own children—of the dangers lurking in grocery aisles and boutiques. When you see the ads on TV and the products on the shelf, you assume they are safe, and in a perfect world they would be.

Once you substitute natural oils for synthetic perfumes, those perfumes slowly cease to appeal to you anymore, and they may even cause headaches. Your nose recognizes synthetic toxins it hadn't noticed when you constantly inhaled them. People tell me all the time how good I smell because now I create unique fragrances with pure essential oils. They do my body good, not harm, while helping me smell fantastic. Let the rich, adaptive fragrance of davana make an excellent top note for a custom fragrance of your own.

Infused Living

Diffuse a few drops davana oil alone or blended with a complementary oil to create a relaxing environment at the end of a busy day. Apply it to your wrists or neck to help you destress.

DIVINELY DAVANA PERFUME BLEND

6 drops lime
6 drops vanilla
4 drops davana
4 drops black spruce
4 drops copaiba
3 drops ylang ylang
3 drops sandalwood

Add davana to facial care products to clear blemishes and nourish skin.

Combine the oils in a 5-ml glass roll-on bottle and top with 80 proof vodka. Shake gently to combine and before each use.

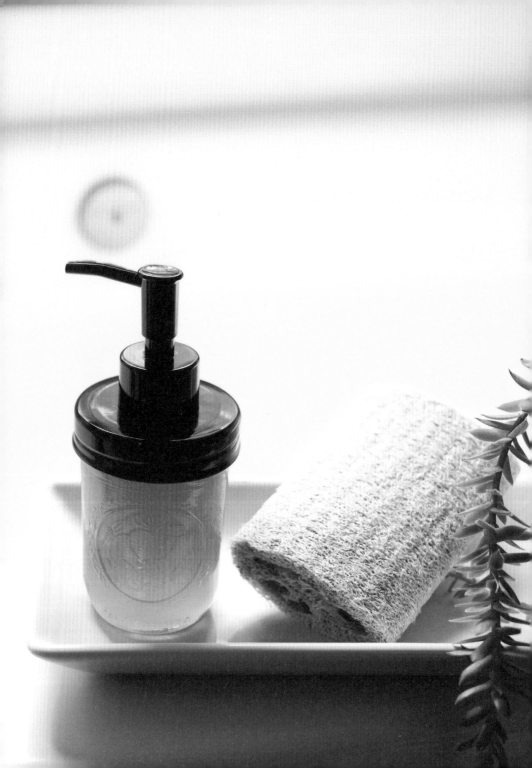

13

ELEMI

The Essentials: *topical, aromatic*

Elemi, also known as Poor Man's Frankincense, performs many of the same functions as its more well-known cousins, frankincense and myrrh, but at a fraction of the cost. It's a great choice for building an oils collection on a budget!

Wisdom from the Garden

Elemi, along with myrrh and frankincense, is a resin-based oil from the *Burseraceae* family with a fascinating history. In Europe, elemi has a long history of use in skin salves and healing ointments. Its resin was sometimes used by artists as an ingredient in varnishes. In the early seventeenth century, a physician used elemi in his practice and on soldiers' battle wounds. Further back, it was used by the Egyptians for embalming. Elemi has been used as an expectorant and for chest and arthritis pain.[1] Incorporate it into your beauty routine for healthy, moisturized skin. Diffuse elemi when you or your children need extra focus or during prayer time. Combine with a carrier oil and massage onto tired muscles.

The fresh, spicy scent of elemi blends well with cinnamon bark, frankincense, myrrh, rosemary, or lavender in the diffuser.

With Intelligent Design

In 2006 I started a web design business within months of starting my blog. I read books on Photoshop and Dreamweaver, programs used for graphics and web development, and jumped in based more on my desire and instinct than my knowledge and experience. It was one of the hardest, scariest, and most amazing things I've ever done. It forced me to learn new skills and languages (HTML and CSS) while using them—the ultimate on-the-job training. Ordinarily I tend to overthink things and, if I'm not careful, only research and never act (analysis paralysis). I'm all about education, but placing more emphasis on training than intuition can squelch creativity and prevent us from taking action. In some circumstances, this would have rewritten history.

Did you realize Frank Sinatra couldn't read music? Neither could Paul McCartney or any of the Beatles for that matter. Johannes Vermeer, one of my favorite painters, registered himself as a master painter with his local guild in the Netherlands when he was 21 years old, but there is no record that he had a master, formal training, or an apprenticeship of any kind. Did he study the work of great artists, use his instincts, and train himself? How different the world would look if Sinatra, McCartney, Vermeer, and many others had been more concerned about what they didn't know than what they did!

It's easy to believe you should know everything about essential oils before you use them, but just like God who created them, their capabilities are vast. I discovered new things every day while researching this book, and I will continue to learn more in the months and years to come. When you read about the characteristics of essential oils, you find many that share the same properties. Multiple oils are anti-inflammatory, antibacterial, antifungal, antiseptic, refreshing to the air and the spirit, help with relaxation and stress relief, improve the condition of skin, help you sleep, relieve pain, and improve digestion or focus. Which ones should you use? It may involve trial and error or personal preference. Different oils may work differently on different people, just as caffeine doesn't affect everyone the same. Everybody and every *body* is unique, and your body knows what to do with essential oils even if you don't understand them. The important thing is to use them. A bottle that sits unopened in a box or on a shelf won't do you any good. God is an intelligent designer, and He created us and plants to work together. Don't squander His gifts. Take powerful, multipurpose oils like elemi, begin to use them, and discover what they can do for you!

Infused Living

Diffuse the powerful combination of elemi, myrrh, and frankincense during prayer time for a sense of clarity, grounding, and focus.

—

DIY BODY WASH ♆

⅔ cup Castile soap

¼ cup honey or agave

1 tsp. vitamin E oil

15 drops elemi

10 drops grapefruit

5 drops geranium

Add elemi to your nighttime skin-care routine for extra moisture.

Place all of the ingredients in an 8-oz. Mason jar with a pump lid. Shake to blend and before each use.

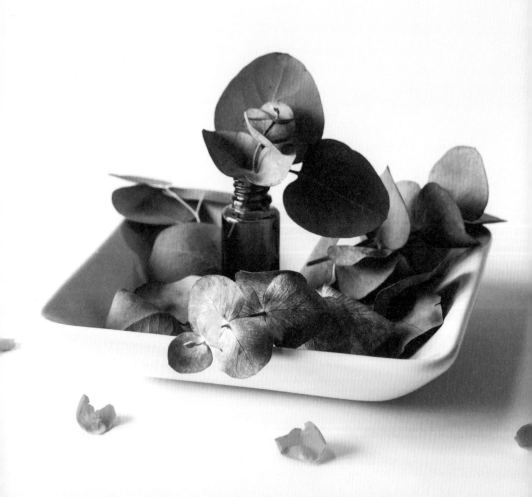

14

EUCALYPTUS

The Essentials: *aromatic, topical*

Eucalyptus was the first oil I purchased beyond my starter kit. I am crazy about its clean, stimulating aroma, and you'll love the way it helps you breathe when you have a cold or congestion, or when exercising.

Wisdom from the Garden

Eucalyptus, steam distilled from the leaves of an evergreen tree native to Australia, has long been used as a cough suppressant and to clear mucous from the chest. Eucalyptus is an anti-inflammatory that can ease cold sore symptoms and joint pain. Because of the oil's antibacterial properties, it can be used for oral care and as an ingredient in natural deodorants.[1] Eucalyptus essential oil and olive oil combine to create a synergy with antimicrobial and wound-healing properties, beneficial for topical application.[2]

The clean, refreshing aroma of eucalyptus blends well with geranium, lemon, lavender, lemongrass, or sandalwood in the diffuser.

Breathe Again

As a child, my mother decorated our home with dried eucalyptus stems. I remember how she dusted and lightly dampened the leaves to freshen and revive their aroma. Even beyond sentimental memories, I've always loved eucalyptus. Before I started using natural essential oils, I bought a eucalyptus-scented lotion that contained synthetic chemicals and fragrance. After a few minutes on my skin, the scent would change and become unpleasant. Thankfully, it discouraged me from using it, and I eventually tossed it in the trash. Our skin is our body's largest organ, and it is designed to protect us. We should protect it too.

I always carry a eucalyptus oil blend in my purse. My son runs cross-country and track and uses eucalyptus topically and aromatically at meets, both inhaling it and rubbing it on his chest. Sometimes we forget and I take it to him at the last minute, right before the race. When that happens, half the team ends up using it. My son is a competitive runner, and I love offering him this safe, effective boost.

Eucalyptus makes a lovely addition to your collection for a multitude of reasons. You'll find yourself reaching for this soothing oil often to open your sinuses or to make your home smell like a spa.

Infused Living

To breathe better or relieve sinus congestion, add a few drops of eucalyptus to steaming water, cover your head with a towel, and then bend over the bowl and breathe in its scent. You can also add it to your diffuser or inhale a drop or two of eucalyptus in your cupped hands.

SOOTHING CHEST RUB 🥄

½ cup grapeseed, coconut, or carrier oil of choice

¼ cup olive oil

¼ cup beeswax pellets

20 drops eucalyptus

20 drops peppermint

> Rub eucalyptus on your chest or the bottom of your feet for respiratory support.

Combine the carrier oil, olive oil, and beeswax in a pan over low heat or in a double boiler. Heat slowly until the beeswax melts. Remove from heat and allow to cool for five minutes. Stir in essential oils and then pour into one 8-oz. or two 4-oz. Mason jars. Cap immediately. The mixture will thicken as it cools. Rub on chest, back, and bottoms of feet for sinus relief. Store at room temperature and use within one year.

HELLO, HANDSOME! COLOGNE BLEND 🥄

10 drops orange

8 drops grapefruit

5 drops eucalyptus

3 drops lime

Add the oils to a 5-ml glass roller bottle and top with 80 proof vodka or a carrier oil (vodka will kill germs; use up blends with carrier oil within a year), or add oils to a 5-ml atomizer and top with 80 proof vodka. Don't be surprised when even strangers mention how good you smell!

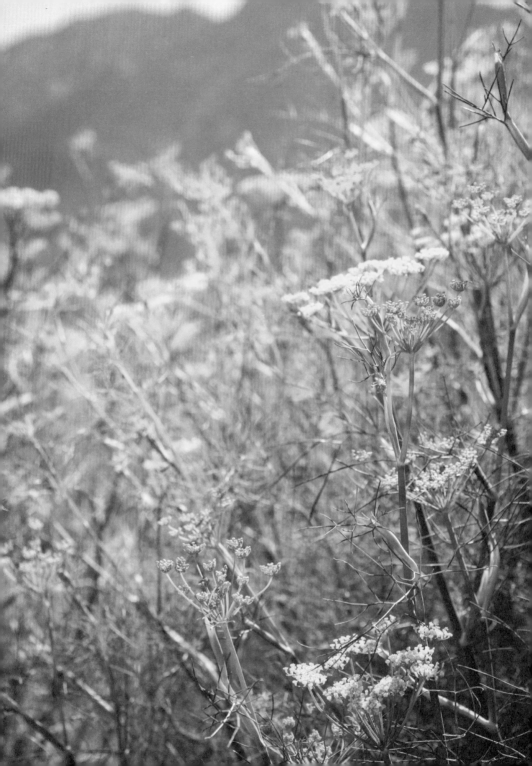

15

FENNEL

The Essentials: *aromatic, topical, internal; avoid during pregnancy or if you have epilepsy*

If you enjoy black licorice, you'll love the sweet taste of fennel oil. It's like a drop of sugar in your mouth that soothes your stomach.

Wisdom from the Garden

Fennel has a rich and fascinating history. In medieval times people believed that when hung over a door, fennel would fend off evil spirits. In Greek mythology, Prometheus stole fire from Mount Olympus, hid it in a stalk of fennel, and gave it to man. Absinthe, a highly alcoholic beverage that was banned in the United States in the early 1900s and reauthorized for sale in 2007, contains fennel along with other botanicals.

The ancient Greek physician Hippocrates, known as "The Founder of Medicine" and credited with creating the Hippocratic Oath, recommended fennel to stimulate milk production in nursing mothers. Women have used it for hundreds of years for that purpose (although it should be used with caution during pregnancy). Fennel oil is steam distilled from the crushed seeds of the fennel plant. Add it to an empty vegetable capsule, as a seasoning in recipes, or to tea for internal consumption, or put a few drops in an empty glass roller bottle and add a carrier oil like coconut to create a topical roll-on. A roll-on with fennel and a carrier oil can also be used to relieve colic or gas in infants.[1]

Fennel oil displays antifungal and antibacterial activities[2] and can aid weight loss by increasing metabolism and serving as an appetite suppressant.[3] Fennel relieves gassiness and constipation and can improve digestion. Aromatically, fennel oil blends well with lavender, lemon, or rosemary in the diffuser.

Self-Defense for Your Gut

Last week I walked into a field of fennel, the plants stretching high above my head. Feathery leaves and small yellow flowers surrounded me as I moved among the dense foliage that created a natural air conditioner, like a cool oasis on a hot day. As a black-thumbed gardener, I was fascinated by both the controlled order and the thriving wildness of these plants. It was a glorious sight.

Originally, I didn't expect to like fennel oil. I had a preconceived notion it would smell and taste icky. When I earned a free bottle, months passed before I even opened it. Now fennel is one of the oils my husband and I rotate in our nightly homemade essential oil capsules. Instead of supporting our digestive system reactively—reaching for an oil that supports it when we experience tummy trouble—we use them proactively to protect our gut health. The balance of good and bad bacteria in that region is important for more than digestion. It's crucial to our hormones, skin, immune systems, and possibly even the treatment and prevention of some diseases.[4] Don't be afraid to embrace fennel the way I was. This aromatic oil with its complex aroma and rich history makes an excellent addition to any oils collection.

Infused Living

Use 1 or 2 drops fennel oil sublingually—under your tongue—when your stomach feels uneasy. Let it sit there for at least 30 seconds before drinking water to wash it down.

TUMMY TROUBLES ROLL-ON

5 drops peppermint

4 drops ginger

3 drops fennel

1 drop lemongrass

Combine the oils in a 10-ml roller bottle and top with a carrier oil, like coconut. Roll on tummies to ease discomfort.

GIRL POWER DIFFUSER BLEND

3 drops fennel

3 drops clary sage

2 drops ginger

> Apply fennel to a cut to fight bacteria and speed healing.

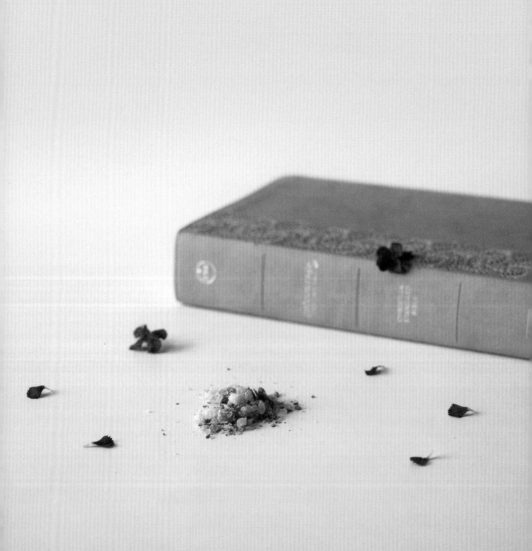

16

FRANKINCENSE

The Essentials: *aromatic, topical, internal*

Whether you spend your days caring for the needs of your children or for those of a large company, we all need a dose of courage from time to time, often from day to day. Frankincense may be just what you need for valor on the go!

Wisdom from the Garden

Frankincense, distilled from the resin of boswellia trees, is also called the Holy Anointing Oil and has been considered a cure-all since Bible times. Used ceremonially by priests in the temple, it was one of the gifts from the three wise men to the baby Jesus, a symbol of His priesthood. This oil can be diffused during prayer time to promote focus. It may help overcome fear, build courage and confidence, improve attitude, and bring about feelings of peace.

———

Be strong and courageous. Do not be afraid or terrified because of them, for the LORD your God goes with you; he will never leave you nor forsake you.

Deuteronomy 31:6 NIV

———

Frankincense oil affects emotional balance, the immune and nervous systems, and the skin, making it an important oil for both mind and body. In ancient times, it was valued more than gold, and only the wealthiest possessed it.

Frankincense blends well in the diffuser with citrus oils such as lemon or grapefruit to energize, or with lavender to relax.

From the Amazing Race to Amazing Grace

The subject line—*The Amazing Race*—immediately caught my eye. Inside, the email began: "Hey there! I work with CBS as a casting producer for *The Amazing Race*! I came across your information online and wanted to reach out because I am looking for competitors for our upcoming season!" I'd heard of *The Amazing Race* but never seen it. My kids, however, were very familiar and went berserk when I shared the email. They were so excited—and even proud of me—that I knew I should consider the request.

The episodes I watched online terrified me. Despite the frightening things I saw (I finally had to quit watching previous episodes), I couldn't resist my kids' excitement and so I sent the following response: "My kids are dying over your email! I will never live it down if I don't follow up with you."

For the next few weeks, I planned for the possibility of being chosen. Preparing to endure physical challenges and confront multiple fears—in a public and fast-paced way—changed how I thought about myself and my health, and I began to make better choices about food and exercise because of what might lie ahead. I even named the memoir I would pen afterwards—*From the Amazing Race to Amazing Grace*—because nothing but the grace of God could carry me through such a thing.

In the end, I wasn't chosen to compete on the show (and honestly, I'm thankful), but it did me good to prepare for it. Contemplating hard things not only forced me to acknowledge my fears and limitations, but it also helped me to remember that the Lord would then, and always, stand beside me through it all.

God doesn't intend for us to walk in fear. In fact, 2 Timothy 1:7 tells us the spirit of fear does not come from Him. Frankincense can help people deal with their everyday fears: taking tests in school, initiating hard conversations, or giving presentations in front of a crowd. I recently saw a friend's anxious daughter apply frankincense before giving a prepared speech in class. Experience had shown her that it helped.

An almost indescribable feeling comes over you when you inhale frankincense: a sense of grounding, clarity, and, yes, an extra dose of courage when you need it most.

Infused Living

Drop frankincense oil into the cupped palm of your hand, breathe in its empowering scent, and then do something you've put off for too long because of fear. Make that call, send that email or text, step outside your comfort zone. If nothing comes of it, you'll know you tried. At least you won't live in fear of it anymore!

FRANKINCENSE, LEMON, AND HONEY FACE MASK

1 tsp. fresh lemon juice

1 tsp. honey

2 drops frankincense

Combine the ingredients and apply to clean skin. Leave on for 20 minutes or more, rinse, and apply your daily moisturizer. Enjoy your velvety smooth skin!

Add frankincense to your facial moisturizer to smooth the appearance of healthy skin and reduce dark spots.

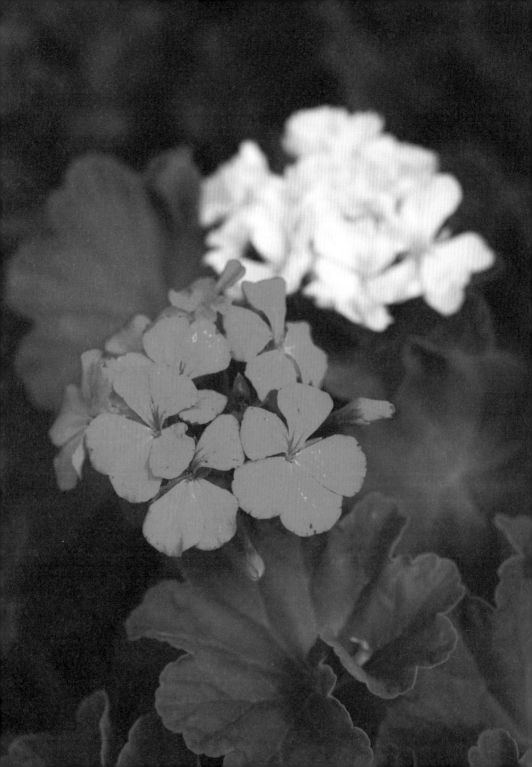

17

GERANIUM

The Essentials: *topical, aromatic*

Looking for a fresh scent to replace toxic perfume chemicals? Geranium, alone or mixed with another essential oil, just might fill the bill! It's one of my favorites to wear on diffuser jewelry, letting its sweet aroma surround me throughout the day.

Wisdom from the Garden

Geranium oil is carefully distilled from a flower native to South Africa. The ancient Egyptians knew of its skin-care benefits. Geranium adds a crisp, floral note to a custom perfume either alone or combined with other essential oils. Add a few drops to your shampoo or conditioner for shinier hair. Geranium oil can improve skin conditions such as acne, aged skin, burns, cellulite, cuts, and eczema, and it can be used to make a DIY deodorant.[1] Geranium oil is a mood booster, stress reducer, and hormone regulator that may be especially helpful for menstruating or menopausal women.[2] One study found aromatherapy massage with geranium oil to ease depression in postmenopausal women.[3]

The sweet scent of geranium diffuses well with lavender, bergamot, citronella, lime, jasmine, orange, or lemon as well as any citrus, floral, or woodsy oil.

In Balance

Sometimes when I walk in my neighborhood I rescue stranded worms on the sidewalk. Many crawl from the grass onto the hot concrete and never make it to the strip of grass on the other side. I don't imagine worms have a strong sense of direction, or a strong sense of anything for that matter. Most of us consider worms to be among the least of all creatures, but still I stop and scoot them back onto the grass to (possibly) live another day. When I think of them, I am reminded of what the Bible says about who is first and who is last:

Many that are first shall be last; and the last shall be first.
Matthew 19:30

God's kingdom is upside down compared to the kingdoms of this world, and at a glance it appears out of balance. The least shall be the greatest (Luke 9:48), our righteousness is as filthy rags (Isaiah 64:6) yet we are children of the King (Galatians 3:26), and His strength is made perfect in our weakness (2 Corinthians 12:9). We know, however, that these seeming contradictions form a divine symmetry.

Geranium oil, too, creates balance. If I had to summarize it in one word, *balance* would be it. Geranium oil helps to balance skin, hair, hormones, and emotions. It calms and grounds me, so I reach for it often and inhale it from the bottle or apply it to my diffuser jewelry. The scent of geranium is gentle yet bold. Because it balances sebum (oil) production, it can benefit all kinds of skin and hair types. I like to blend a drop of geranium oil with a carrier oil such as grapeseed and apply it to my face and neck. Geranium oil can help reduce stress and bring about a sense of peace, effects which are especially helpful for women during their periods or navigating menopause. That may be why I like it so much.

Infused Living

Add 1 or 2 drops geranium oil to your moisturizer. It will not only brighten your skin but help balance your hormones and emotions too. It's an incredible oil for self-care.

HOT FLASH MENOPAUSE COOLING SPRAY

20 drops geranium
20 drops clary sage
10 drops peppermint

Combine the oils in a 2-oz. glass spray bottle and top with witch hazel. Shake to combine and before use. Spray to your neck, arms, and torso when the heat is on!

Rub geranium oil on your abdomen to ease PMS symptoms.

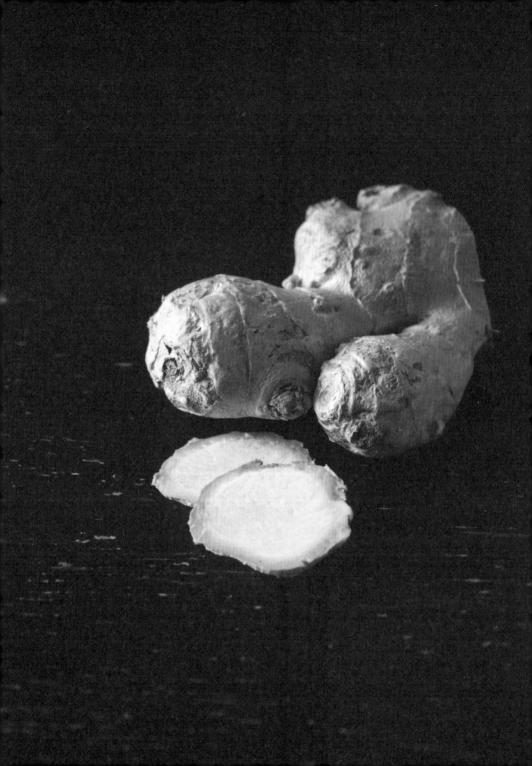

18

GINGER

The Essentials: *aromatic, topical, internal*

There is a reason people drink ginger ale when they have an upset stomach or feel nauseated. Ginger is a potent aid to our digestive systems!

Wisdom from the Garden

Spicy ginger oil, distilled from the root of the ginger plant, gives gingerbread cookies their sweet taste and aroma. It's also a staple in Asian cuisine. Ginger oil can replace fresh ginger in recipes, but because of its concentration you may only need a drop or two. Ginger aids digestion and has been used in natural medicine for thousands of years. Inhaling ginger essential oil helps control nausea[1] and relax airways, which could benefit those with asthma.[2] Its anti-inflammatory[3] and antioxidant properties[4] can benefit us as we age.

The warm, spicy aroma of ginger blends well with citrus oils like lemon, bergamot, and orange; florals like geranium and ylang ylang, or earthy scents like frankincense and eucalyptus in the diffuser.

Ginger to the Rescue!

I met my future husband the final month of my senior year of high school, and I fell hard. Hard. I'd been accepted to an East Coast Ivy League school 1,800 miles from my hometown in Arkansas, and I thought my future was mapped out and firmly under my control. (Feel free to roll your eyes along with me.) By the time I arrived in New Hampshire for my freshman year, I was not only head over heels in love but had abandoned my plan to become a psychiatrist. Biology lab made me squeamish, so medical school didn't sound like a fit after all. (Interestingly enough, I've taught a biology lab for high schoolers once a week for the past decade; however, they're the ones handling the critters.)

We know emotions affect our bodies. Have you ever received news so devastating it made you feel nauseated or as though you had been punched in the gut? Or have you been released from a fear or worry you carried and the sense of relief was almost tangible? Although we may casually throw around the word *lovesick*, it can be real. I spent that freshman fall in a case of digestive distress, gassy and miserable. The longing in my heart did a number on my stomach too.

Years later, during the pregnancies when I experienced the most nausea (I have eight biological children from eight separate pregnancies), I sought relief wherever I could find it: wearing acupressure wrist bands, eating saltine crackers, and drinking ginger ale stronger than the typical grocery store variety. Unfortunately, I began to associate the smell of ginger with nausea, and sometimes this made it worse. The beauty of essential oils that are safe for internal consumption is the ability to add them to a veggie capsule and swallow like a pill. You can inhale ginger oil straight from the bottle for nausea, rub it topically on the stomach area after eating, or add a couple drops to herbal tea for relief. It's a primary component in an oil blend that I don't leave home without because of its ability to quickly help my stomach. Ginger essential oil can come to the rescue when you experience nausea, digestive discomfort, muscle pain, and more.

Infused Living

Combine a few drops ginger essential oil with a carrier oil to create a massage oil, and let ginger's anti-inflammatory properties help soothe your muscle pain.

CLEAR YOUR HEAD ROLL-ON

8 drops ginger
5 drops peppermint
4 drops eucalyptus
3 drops copaiba
2 drops frankincense

Combine the oils in a 10-ml glass roller bottle and top with the carrier oil of your choice. Apply to chest when congested.

WHAT'S COOKING?

3 drops ginger
2 drops clove
2 drops cinnamon bark
1 drop lemon

Inhale ginger oil directly from the bottle to combat nausea.

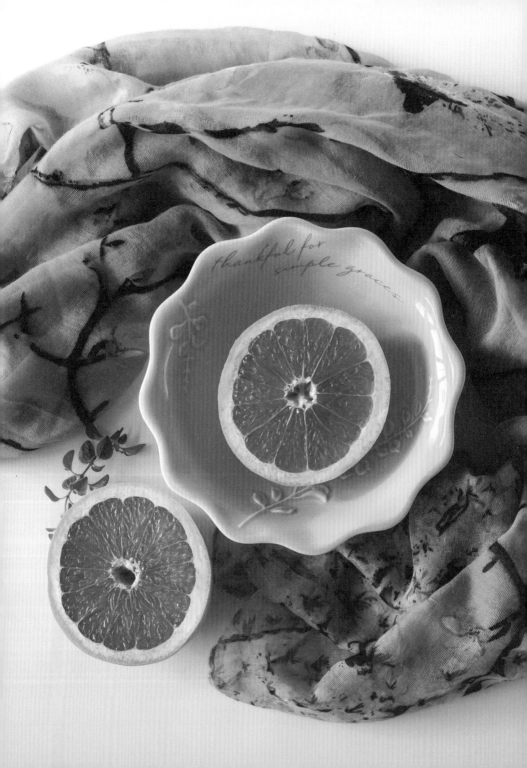

19

GRAPEFRUIT

The Essentials: *topical, aromatic, internal, photosensitive*

Fresh, invigorating grapefruit is a favorite thanks to its sweet, citrusy taste and bright, uplifting scent either in the diffuser or DIY perfume blends. Grapefruit, as well as most citrus oils, is photosensitive, so don't use it on skin that will be exposed to the sun for the next day.

Wisdom from the Garden

Grapefruit oil, cold pressed from the rind of the fruit, may suppress appetite, promote weight loss,[1] and encourage joy and playfulness with its sunny scent. It possesses a wide spectrum of antimicrobial activities.[2] Because of its antibacterial and skin-cleansing properties, grapefruit may promote healthy skin and help in the treatment of acne. Inhaling it activates sympathetic nerve activity and helps activate enzymes in the body that break down fat, resulting in a suppression of weight gain.[3] Although grapefruit juice can affect some medications, grapefruit oil comes from the peel of the fruit. In her book *The Essential Oil Truth: The Facts Without the Hype*, author Jen O'Sullivan says that there is no proof or cited reference of a similar "grapefruit juice effect" from grapefruit essential oil but recommends you consult your doctor before making changes in your regimen because everyone is different.[4]

Uplifting, citrusy grapefruit blends well with basil, bergamot, juniper, lavender, and ylang ylang in the diffuser.

The Dieter's Friend

My body settled into what I eventually termed my life weight in the eighth grade and maintained it for more than 20 years. With my first six pregnancies I gained the weight, nursed it off, and then settled back into that exact weight once my babies were weaned. After the last two pregnancies, in my late thirties, the number increased by three pounds. Now I'm 20 pounds over that. Age (and many hours sitting in a chair writing) is not always kind, especially when it comes to hormones and metabolism. I never gave my weight a thought growing up, but now I think about it every day. It can feel as out of my control as the weather or the stars in the night sky. It used to be so easy.

Grapefruit has been nicknamed the dieter's friend with its ability to reduce appetite, boost metabolism, and contribute to weight loss. The combination of grapefruit, orange, lemon, and patchouli, when inhaled, has been found to suppress appetite by reducing awareness of or desire for food.[5] I have always loved the smell and taste of grapefruit and enjoy it both in my water and in the diffuser. Thankfully, while writing this book I've managed to maintain and even lose a little weight. I tend to gain as much as ten pounds with each book because of the sedentary nature of writing, and it gets harder and harder to lose. If you, too, find the pounds don't slip off as easily as they once did and your weight seems difficult to control, grapefruit may be an excellent oil to add to your collection.

Infused Living

Grapefruit combined with caffeine has been found to tighten the skin and reduce the appearance of cellulite. Fight cellulite with the DIY grapefruit and caffeine body scrub below.

GRAPEFRUIT AND COFFEE CELLULITE SCRUB

1 cup coffee grounds (fresh or used)

½ cup olive or another carrier oil

10 drops grapefruit

5 drops cypress

Combine all ingredients in a glass jar with a lid. Store in the shower and rub this scrub into the skin of your thighs, arms, or wherever you discover dimpled skin. Rinse and repeat a few times a week.

MY SWEET SUMMER

3 drops grapefruit

3 drops orange

1 drop geranium

1 drop blue spruce

Add grapefruit both to your water and to your diffuser as an appetite suppressant.

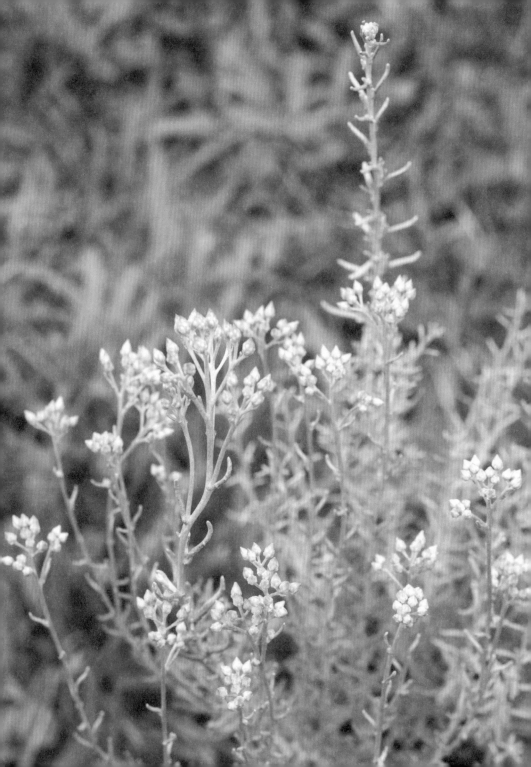

20

HELICHRYSUM

The Essentials: *aromatic, topical, internal*

I've heard the name of this oil pronounced at least three different ways, but no matter how you say it, helichrysum is a healing powerhouse. My family uses a DIY helichrysum-based salve to soothe skin and help with scarring.

Wisdom from the Garden

Helichrysum is steam distilled from the tiny flowers of a plant in the same family as the sunflower and daisy. While those flowers may be common, this oil is a rare prize; good quality helichrysum oil costs about a dollar a drop. Helichrysum, also called "Immortelle" or "everlasting," is known for its regenerative and age-defying benefits. Topically it can be used for acne, infections, burns, scarring, eczema, and wounds,[1] and has proven antibacterial[2] and anti-inflammatory[3] properties. Helichrysum may be helpful for headaches[4] and respiratory complaints.

While helichrysum has a sweet, fruity flavor that blends well with geranium, lavender, clary sage, or citrus oils in the diffuser, I would save it for topical application.

When You Need to Heal

When I work on a book, I tend to listen to the same musician or even the same album over and over, as if the project has its own soundtrack. Eventually it becomes a conditioned response. The music puts me in the headspace to work. While writing this book's proposal—a document designed to persuade a publisher that its concept is marketable and people will buy it (thank you for doing so, by the way)—I listened to the group NEEDTOBREATHE, who were new to me. I always thought I would like them, and it turns out I do. The song "Happiness" summarizes feelings I have about my goals, business, life as a writer, and family almost better than I could. Shortly after I finished the book proposal, we saw NEEDTOBREATHE in concert. It was a perfect culmination to the work—a bow tied around the proposal process—and I paused the needle on NEEDTOBREATHE, saving them for the period of book writing if a publisher accepted my proposal.

And then I discovered satellite radio.

After an oil change, my car dealership offered to activate my SUV with two free months of SiriusXM, no strings attached, no credit card required. It was a wise marketing move. I've become so attached to the Beatles Channel and '80s on 8 that I'll be a lifetime subscriber. My children think I should just play Spotify from my phone, but I'm hooked on the programming, the interviews, and the fascinating tidbits I learn on satellite radio. Where else will I hear backstories for the songs straight from the mouths of John, Paul, George, and Ringo? I jokingly call this my Beatles immersion period. Writing can be solitary, lonely work, but "Good Day Sunshine," "Penny Lane," and "Oh! Darling" kept me company, drifting from my speakers and through my brain, day by day as this book continued to take shape. Songs like "Blackbird," "In My Life," and "Let it Be" speak to us. The lyrics break and then heal us.

Just as music can help heal our hearts, oils can help heal our bodies. I have no doubt God provided them for that purpose. I'm not sure how to say helichrysum, but I choose to give it a long ē sound, like heal, for all the ways it helps our bodies. If your body and spirit need healing, you might need a Beatles immersion and a bottle of helichrysum of your own.

Infused Living

Add 2 drops helichrysum to a carrier oil and create a massage oil after heavy exercise. Play music that allows your mind to unwind as well as your body.

HEALING SALVE

7 T. grapeseed, almond, jojoba, extra virgin olive, or sunflower oil

1 to 2 T. beeswax pellets

10 drops helichrysum

10 drops geranium

10 drops lavender

10 drops frankincense

10 drops copaiba

4-oz. Mason jar

> Use helichrysum after an injury for pain relief and to reduce bruising.

Combine the base carrier oil and beeswax in a pan over low heat or in a double boiler. Warm until the beeswax melts (which may be longer than you think), and then remove from heat and allow to cool for 5 minutes. Stir in the essential oils and then pour into a 4-oz. Mason jar, capping the jar immediately. The mixture will thicken as it cools. Store at room temperature and use within one year.

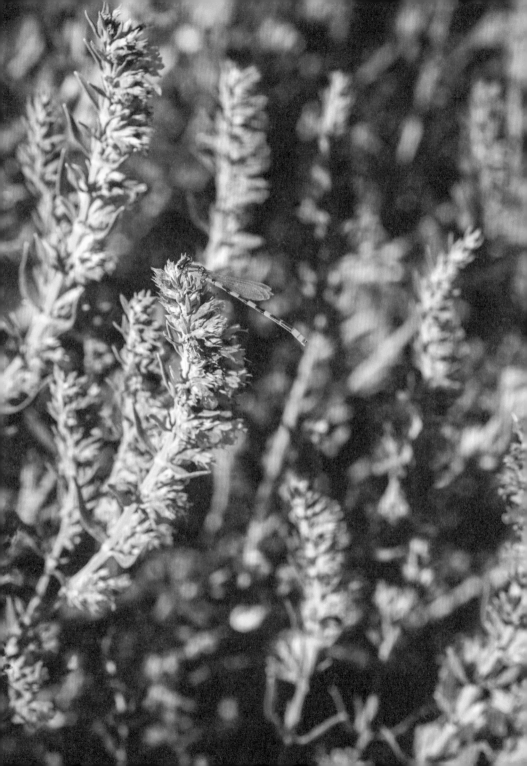

21

HYSSOP

The Essentials: *aromatic, topical, internal; avoid during pregnancy, for children under two, or if you have epilepsy*

Hyssop has been used medicinally since biblical times and is mentioned 12 times in the Bible. Add it to your oils collection to incorporate ancient wisdom into your modern lifestyle.

Wisdom from the Garden

Hyssop, steam distilled from the leaves and stems of the plant, possesses valuable antioxidant properties, has antimicrobial properties[1] effective against bacterial multiresistance,[2] and makes a strong antiseptic.

Historically, hyssop was used for spiritual cleansing, to help focus the mind for prayer and meditation, for respiratory relief, and as a decongestant. In modern times, it has been used to ease anxiety, arthritis, asthma, respiratory infections, sore throats, cuts and wounds, and for detoxification and emotional balance.[3]

The warm, pungent scent of hyssop blends well with clary sage, fennel, geranium, sage, and citrus in the diffuser.

Cleansing and Freedom

During the exodus from Egypt, Moses instructed the elders of Israel to dip a bunch of the hyssop plant in the blood of a Passover lamb, strike the top and side posts of the door frame with it, and not leave the house until morning as protection from the plague of death. In the night, the Egyptians perished, but the Hebrews were spared. They were told to observe this ordinance forever, both as a reminder to them and as an opportunity to tell their children of God's provision and how He delivered them safely from Egyptian bondage (Exodus 12:21-27). The strong, slightly sweet smell of hyssop would create a powerful aromatic reminder of freedom, cleansing, and God's protection.

At the cross, Jesus spoke the words, "I thirst," to fulfill the prophecy of Psalm 69:21, and a sponge soaked in vinegar was lifted to His lips on a stalk of the hyssop plant, just before He spoke the words "It is finished." (John 19:28-30). In the Old Testament hyssop represented cleansing and freedom, and at the cross we were cleansed and freed by the blood of Jesus Christ—with the aroma of hyssop and blood in the air.

———

Purge me with hyssop, and I shall be clean: wash me,
and I shall be whiter than snow.

Psalm 51:7

———

Infused Living

To help prevent bruising and reduce immediate swelling, apply hyssop to a cold compress or a cloth wrapped around an ice bag, and place on the injury site.

DIY ANTIMICROBIAL COUNTERTOP CLEANER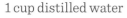

1 cup distilled water

1 cup white vinegar

10 drops hyssop

10 drops clove

10 drops orange

Combine the oils, water, and vinegar in a 16-oz. glass spray bottle. Shake to combine and before using with a microfiber cloth to clean countertops.

WELLNESS DIFFUSER BLEND

5 drops hyssop

3 drops frankincense

2 drops eucalyptus

2 drops tea tree

Diffuse hyssop to stimulate creativity.

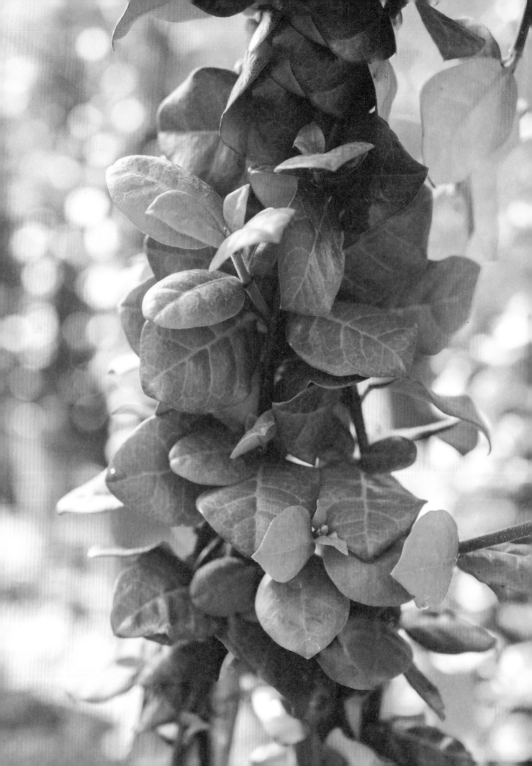

22

JASMINE

The Essentials: *aromatic, topical, internal*

Searching for a natural alternative to toxin-filled commercial perfumes? The lovely, exotic scent of jasmine oil may be exactly what you seek!

Wisdom from the Garden

Jasmine is one of the most expensive essential oils because it is difficult to obtain. The flowers of the jasmine plant, part of the olive family, must be picked in the dark hours of night, and more than 10 pounds of them are required to produce a 5-ml bottle of oil. The delicate flowers cannot be steam distilled, so jasmine is technically an absolute or essence rather than a true essential oil.

The uplifting scent of jasmine affects emotions. This powerful anti-depressant can reduce anxiety, relieve depression, and lift your mood.[1] Researchers have found jasmine to be "as calming as valium," delivering the same benefits as sedatives, sleeping pills, and relaxants without their serious potential side effects.[2] Use jasmine in conjunction with prayer, but don't hesitate to seek medical help for severe depression.

Jasmine's exotic floral scent makes a lovely cologne and produces feelings of confidence in the wearer. Its fragrance may have an aphrodisiac effect and has been referred to as the "queen of the night" and the "moonlight of the grove." It can be beneficial for skin care[3] and has a stimulating effect when combined with a carrier oil for a massage.

Jasmine's sweet scent blends well with frankincense, geranium, lemongrass, or spearmint in the diffuser.

Sweet Jasmine

I love to jog on our county's beautiful greenway system during my kids' cross-country and track practices. The lovely, wooded pathways provide a pleasant distraction from the burn in my legs and the shortness of my breath. Sometimes I pass people from behind or as we travel in opposite directions, and I catch fascinating snippets of conversation, like a fly on the wall. One morning I overheard one walker say to another, "Everything is sadder in the night. More dire," and I recognized the truth in these words. How many times have I gone to bed with the weight of the world on my shoulders only to awake to a fresh, new day?

———

His anger endureth but a moment; in his favour is life:
weeping may endure for a night, but joy cometh in the morning.
Psalm 30:5

———

When my kids were little, my patience and stamina lasted only until my husband got home from work. He spent time with the kids and took on bathing and bedtime duties so I could have some quiet, adult time, even if that simply meant time alone in the kitchen. Parents experience the joys and sorrows, the successes and failures, the magnificent and mundane moments of their children's lives. Because we are emotionally invested, they can elevate our mood or pull us down. It's human nature to proclaim the good but hide the bad. If you see a child who's struggling, chances are there's a mother struggling too.

Because essential oils reach our limbic system, they affect our emotions in powerful ways. They can be indispensable agents when used to enhance our emotional well-being. Jasmine is a lovely oil that can help reduce anxiety and lift your mood. Although I like to inhale it from the bottle, this doesn't compare to the experience of wearing it on my wrist or neck. Jasmine blends with my body chemistry and creates an even more incredible smell. I remember the first time I put a drop on my wrist; I couldn't stop smelling it. I felt wonderful. Now it's a key component in an oil blend I carry with me and wear as perfume. Multifaceted jasmine can boost your mood, ease your mind, or make you feel beautiful and confident. Its name comes from the Persian word *yasmin*, meaning "a gift from God," and I believe that it is. Jasmine is one of my favorite oils, and I think you'll love the way it affects you too.

Infused Living

Do you have a friend or acquaintance who is going through a difficult season? Check in this week and offer a word of encouragement and, if possible, some uplifting oils. Two drops of frankincense, one drop of lemon, and two drops of jasmine make a cheerful combination in the diffuser.

FEELS LIKE SPRING

2 drops jasmine
2 drops geranium
2 drops ylang ylang
2 drops frankincense

Diffuse jasmine oil to relax and unwind after a long day.

SUMMER DIFFUSER RECIPES

INTO THE WOODS

7 drops blue spruce

2 drops cypress

1 drop wintergreen

1 drop bergamot

FRESH AIR

3 drops eucalyptus

3 drops pine

2 drops lemon

2 drops lime

2 drops orange

SPA DAY

4 drops lemon

3 drops lavender

SUMMER BREEZE

3 drops tangerine

1 drop spearmint

1 drop bergamot

COASTAL BLISS

2 drops cedarwood

2 drops frankincense

2 drops orange

1 drop rosemary

CITRUS FRESH

2 drops orange

2 drops tangerine

2 drops grapefruit

2 drops lemon

1 drop spearmint

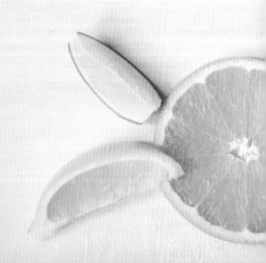

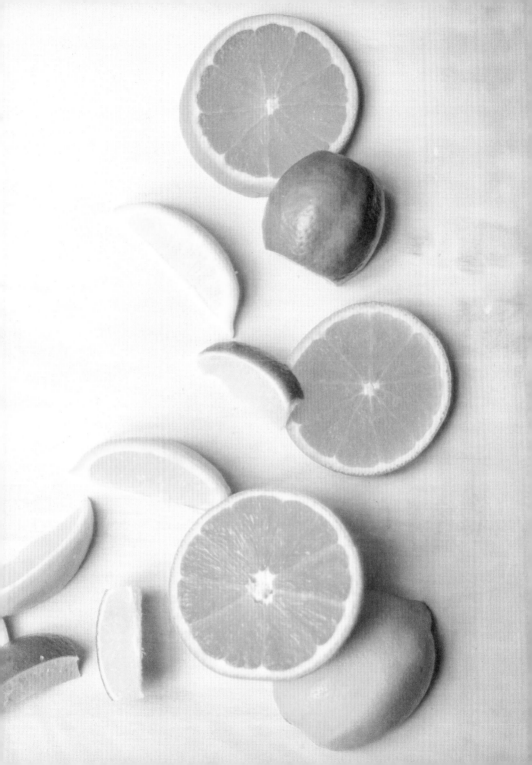

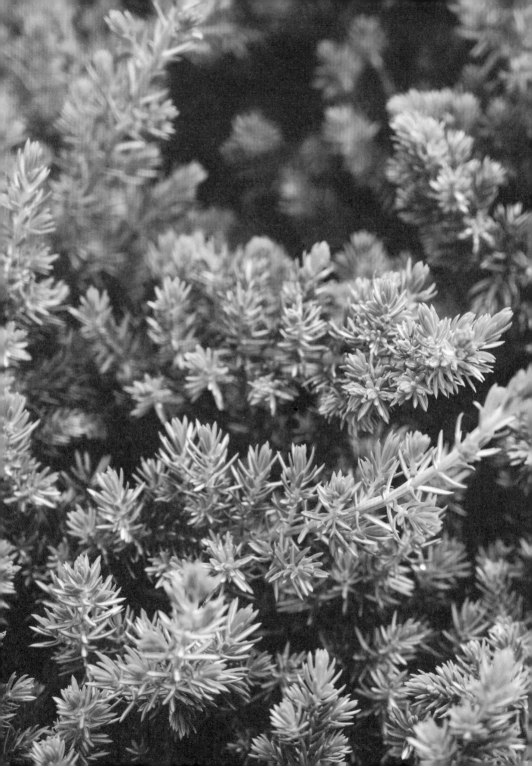

23

JUNIPER

The Essentials: *aromatic, topical, internal; avoid for children under two*

Sweet, earthy juniper oil cleanses both body and spirit and can help evoke feelings of peace. This emotionally uplifting oil with solid physical benefits makes a wonderful addition to your oils collection.

Wisdom from the Garden

Steam distilled from the stems, leaves, and flowers of the evergreen shrub/small tree, juniper has a rich history. Ancient Egyptian doctors recommended it as a laxative. Native Americans used juniper berries to assist with childbirth and to treat infections, arthritis, and wounds. Juniper has been used for gas, indigestion, warts, respiratory problems, and back pain, and the berries were eaten to freshen bad breath.[1] Because burning juniper branches seemed to ward off contagious diseases, medieval physicians chewed the berries while treating patients and burned the branches in hospitals. The French returned to this practice in World War II, burning juniper in hospitals as an antiseptic when their drug supply ran low.[2]

Juniper is known for its skin-soothing properties,[3] making it beneficial for itchy conditions such as poison ivy and psoriasis and to support a healthy complexion. It can relieve burns, help to heal wounds, prevent infection and scarring, and soothe inflammation.[4] Juniper can ease tension and relieve muscle spasms.[5] Chemical compounds found in the oil have antiobesity and antioxidant properties. When used topically, juniper oil may reduce water retention.[6] As a powerful diuretic with antiseptic properties, juniper supports the urinary system.[7] Juniper berries are the predominant flavor in the alcoholic drink gin.

The crisp, woodsy scent of juniper blends well with bergamot, cypress, geranium, lavender, tea tree, rosemary, and all citrus oils in the diffuser.

Oils and Emotions

To my logical mind, initially it was easier to see how oils could benefit us more physically than emotionally. If you apply an oil to something that hurts and then it feels better, that's simple cause and effect. My husband and I have had measurable results from taking oils internally, verified by bloodwork. That, too, is easy to see.

Although feelings may be harder to quantify, essential oils can do amazing things for our mood and outlook. For many, the emotional effects are life changing. Juniper oil has long been used to help evoke feelings of peace and spiritual awareness. It can help us deal with stress and anxiety. Because of their calming and stabilizing effects on our emotions, mood, and stress level, oils like juniper can help us deal with difficulties or traumas we'd rather ignore, allowing us to heal emotionally and mentally. Juniper, as well as bergamot, can decrease our blood pressure and heart rate; together, they create a relaxing yet uplifting diffuser combination.

As you continue to use essential oils, you will discover how they affect you and your family emotionally, and you will learn how to use your diffuser to influence the atmosphere in your home. Essential oils that come from trees can be grounding. When life and circumstances feel out of control, bend your knees in prayer and then reach for a stabilizing oil like juniper.

The peace of God, which transcends all understanding,
will guard your hearts and your minds in Christ Jesus.
Philippians 4:7 NIV

Infused Living

Aromatherapy massage has proven emotional benefits. Blend juniper with a carrier oil for an aromatherapy massage oil to destress your day.

HEADACHE HELPER ROLL-ON

6 drops lavender
6 drops eucalyptus
6 drops peppermint
3 drops lemon
2 drops juniper
2 drops basil

Combine the essential oils in a 15-ml roller bottle and top with your carrier oil of choice. Shake gently to combine. Roll on temples, forehead, or back of the neck as needed.

Add a few drops of juniper to Epsom salt for a relaxing, spalike bath.

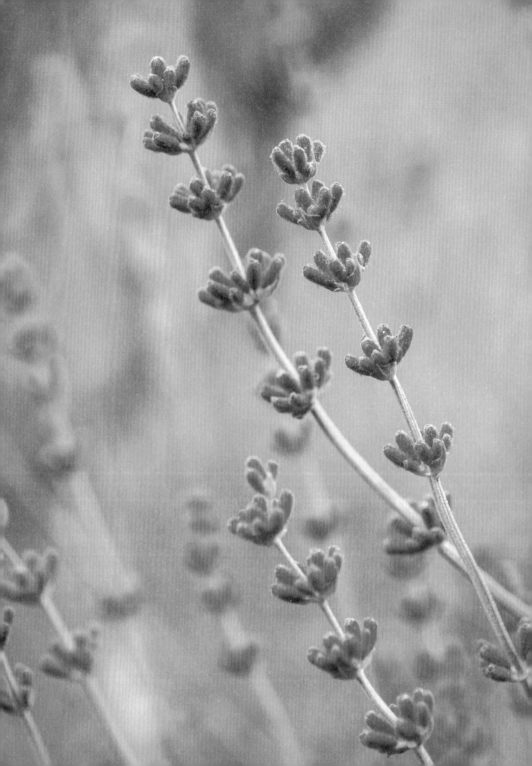

24

LAVENDER

The Essentials: *aromatic, topical, internal*

Did you know lavender is the world's most popular essential oil? It's called the Swiss Army knife of essential oils because it combines so many beneficial properties into one amazingly awesome oil!

Wisdom from the Garden

Lavender oil, steam distilled from the flowering tops of the plant, was as popular in the past as it is today. When King Tutankhamen's tomb was entered in 1923, the faint scent of lavender, used in Egyptian embalming, could be detected after 3,000 years. Cleopatra was said to have used it to lure Julius Caesar and Mark Antony. Dioscorides, a Greek botanist and physician, wrote about the healing benefits of lavender. So did German abbess Hildegard of Bingen, considered to be the first herbalist. When French chemist René-Maurice Gattefossé badly burned his hands in his laboratory in 1910, he rolled on a grassy lawn to extinguish them and then rinsed them with lavender oil. The results impressed him greatly, and the oil possibly saved his life. He went on to publish the 1937 book *Aromathérapie*, the first use of the word *aromatherapy*.

Lavender can heal damaged skin; speed tissue regeneration; and treat burns, sunburns, insect bites, bee stings, and wounds.[1] Tests have found lavender helps those suffering from anxiety or postpartum depression.[2] Lavender oil can reduce stress, improve your mood, and help you relax and sleep better.

If you've tried lavender-scented products in the past and didn't like the smell, give a quality, therapeutic-grade lavender oil a try. Because of lavender's popularity, many products on the market contain synthetic additives or use solvents to stretch the plant yield. Lavender oil altered in this way does not have the same aroma or benefits as pure lavender essential oil.

Lavender blends well with geranium, rosemary, clary sage, and citrus oils. Lavender combined equally with lemon and peppermint is known as LLP, or the Allergy Bomb, for its ability to relieve seasonal allergies.

Good Night, Sleep Tight

Lavender was the first bottle I emptied of the 11 in my essential oils starter kit. I joined an oils company at a time when I was under a lot of stress professionally and personally. My first book released and I turned in my second within a month of each other, and two of our sons were getting married three weeks and a day apart, both out of state. Sometimes I rebel against the rules—and there were so many of them!—but that wasn't an option as the mother of the groom(s). I needed to arrange rehearsal dinners, dress myself in the appropriate style and color, and coordinate clothing, fittings, and alterations for my family too.

At the end of each long, demanding day, I'd lie down in bed and reach for my bottle of lavender, rub a drop or two together in my palms, and cup my hands over my nose to inhale the intoxicating scent. It seeped straight into my brain and signaled peace to my overworked mind. I remember the day I told my husband, "I never want to be without this lavender again."

I also remember the night I shook and shook my little bottle and declared that the reducer must be clogged. "You use it every night in the dark. Maybe it's empty," my husband replied. Oh, my word—it was! That week I learned two valuable lessons: 1) remove the reducer in the top of the bottle to access the last few precious drops, and 2) keep a close eye on the volume of your favorite oils.

The limbic system, the part of our brain responsible for our sense of smell, is tied to emotion and memory. I shared earlier how the scent of a particular lotion still brings back childhood memories of my mother, and a particular brand of baby shampoo reminds me of my kids when they were small, so it's not surprising to associate the smell of lavender with feelings of rest and calm. Instead of over-the-counter sleeping pills, I now rely on a travel diffuser and my trusty bottle of lavender when I leave home. Good night, sleep tight.

Infused Living

Try lavender by itself or blended with orange or cedarwood in your diffuser tonight for a good night's sleep, and train your brain to let go and relax in response to its heavenly scent.

DIY SUNBURN SPRAY

⅓ cup liquid aloe vera juice
10 drops lavender essential oil
10 drops peppermint essential oil
Olive oil

> Add a drop of lavender to mascara to condition lashes.

Combine the essential oils and aloe vera juice in a 4-oz. glass spray bottle and top with olive oil. For cooling relief, spray on skin that's spent too much time in the sun.

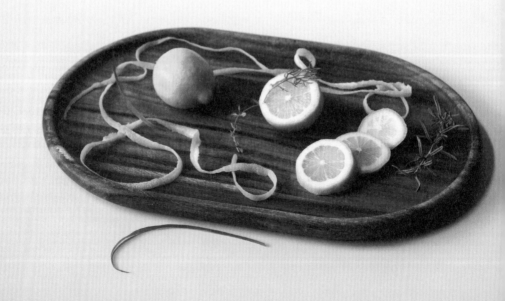

25

LEMON

The Essentials: *aromatic, topical, internal, photosensitive*

If you have trouble waking up in the morning or feel glum when winter's chill keeps you indoors, the bright, cheerful aroma of lemon oil may be just what you need, fresh like a sunny summer's day.

Wisdom from the Garden

Lemon essential oil is cold pressed from the rind of the fruit and more concentrated than lemon juice. Used in a variety of skin-care and cleaning products, lemon oil cleanses while its fresh aroma invigorates. Substitute lemon oil for lemon juice—add just a drop or two—in both sweet and savory recipes. Citrus fragrances have been found to boost immunity and lift depression. Lemon oil is rich in limonene, a chemical found in the peels of citrus fruits and known for its incredible health benefits. Research has found lemon oil to effectively reduce stress too. [1]

The warm, fresh smell of lemon blends well in the diffuser with florals like geranium, rose, and ylang ylang; with citrus scents like grapefruit, lime, and orange; or with just about anything: eucalyptus, frankincense, juniper, rosemary, or tea tree. Equal parts lemon, lavender, and peppermint are particularly effective against allergies.

Lemony Fresh

I've always found lemon's scent and taste irresistible. Lemon enhances the flavor of my sweet tea and the smell of my cleaning products. Not only is lemon one of my family's most-loved essential oils—and my teen son's favorite—but it's readily available and inexpensive too.

Because lemon effectively cleans skin and fights acne, my teens apply it to their faces after washing, but I offer you the same warning I give them: Lemon oil may cause sun sensitivity, so avoid using it on skin that will be exposed to the sun. Lemon is one of the oils I sometimes add to my nighttime skin-care products for younger-looking skin.

Remember using lemon juice mixed with water on your hair as a teen? Mix a drop of lemon oil with water and spritz on your hair before a day in the sun for natural highlights. Just don't get lemon in your eyes!

One of my favorite things about essential oils that are safe for human consumption is the convenience. I tend to either let fruit go bad before I use it or forget to buy what I need when I need it. (Meal planning isn't one of my greatest strengths.) Keeping culinary oils on hand enables me to have lemon's delightfully refreshing flavor available whether I remember to pick up lemons at the grocery store or not.

You've probably heard that lemon juice can damage the enamel on your teeth because of its high-acidic content, but lemon essential oil is easier on your teeth and stomach. Cold pressed from the lemon rind and extremely concentrated, it takes 75 lemons to make one 15-ml bottle of lemon essential oil. Lemon oil in my morning water is a powerful detox. Sometimes I add a drop of lemon to my toothpaste for extra whitening, fresh breath, and simply because I love its flavor. (Remember to use internally only the highest-quality oils labeled safe for human consumption.)

Lemon's fresh scent makes it particularly appealing in the diffuser. Diffusing lemon can not only reduce household odors but also perk up your people and put a smile on your face.

Infused Living

Use lemon oil to remove the sticky residue left behind after removing price tags or the labels on your empty essential oil bottles. Add a drop of lemon oil to plain or vanilla yogurt. Diffuse lemon oil to add a little sunshine to your day!

——

LEMON DUSTING SPRAY AND FURNITURE POLISH

1 cup distilled water

¼ cup vinegar (to cut through grease and grime)

2 tsp. olive oil (shines and protects wood)

10 to 15 drops lemon

Combine all ingredients in a 16-oz. glass spray bottle. Shake well before each use. Spray furniture and wipe with a microfiber cloth.

> Lemon oil can break down plastic, so only add lemon oil to beverages in a glass or stainless-steel container.

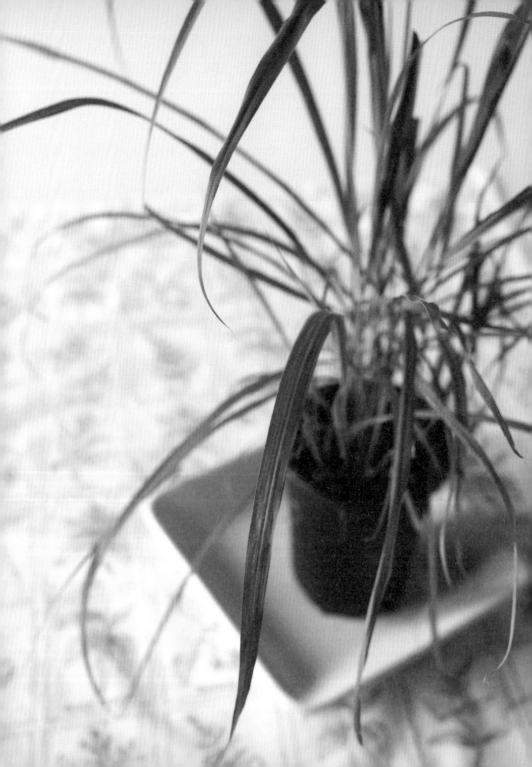

26

LEMONGRASS

The Essentials: *aromatic, topical, internal, hot*

Fresh, citrusy lemongrass is invigorating in the air, powerful on the body, and flavorful in the kitchen. Be sure to add this incredible multipurpose oil to your collection!

Wisdom from the Garden

Lemongrass is distilled from the leaves and woody stalks of the lemongrass plant. Not only does it smell fresh and clean, but it's a powerful oil that works as an anti-inflammatory,[1] can lower cholesterol,[2] and effectively fights antibiotic-resistant bacteria (MRSA).[3] Author Jen O'Sullivan describes essential oils as the pheromones of the plant and insect world because of their ability to attract or repel.[4] Lemongrass oil attracts bees but repels mosquitoes (and we all want to repel mosquitoes, right?). Lemongrass oil can aid your digestion while it flavors your food.

The bright, lemony smell of lemongrass blends well with basil, bergamot, lime, cypress, eucalyptus, geranium, or lavender in the diffuser.

A Life-Changing Oil

We call lemongrass my husband's signature oil. Whatever his problem is, lemongrass seems to be the answer. It was his "aha moment," his "these really do work" oil. I watched him suffer with plantar fasciitis in one foot for about nine months. He'd get out of bed each morning and hobble to the bathroom, pain evident from his groans and the look on his face. He suffered during the day too, but mornings were the worst. Bryan has always been a runner, and thankfully he was able to continue, but the pain afterward was so severe he began to run less often. Now I automatically pull out an oils reference guide or app when we're faced with a problem, but we were new oilers then and didn't immediately try them at the time. When I finally thought to research oils for plantar fasciitis, a web search recommended lemongrass.

I joked that Bryan smelled like a lemon drop when he came to bed that first night. The next morning the difference was almost shocking: serious, marked improvement after months with no relief. I put lemongrass and a carrier oil in a glass bottle with a roll-on applicator, and he applied it to his foot and ankle both morning and night. He used it for only a couple of weeks before the pain was gone.

Once when my shoulder hurt, I applied lemongrass neat (straight and undiluted) at bedtime and woke up without shoulder pain but with a bright red rash in its place. My husband applies it undiluted with no problem, but it's a hot oil for me, and I use it with a generous amount of carrier oil. Lemongrass is an incredible anti-inflammatory that we turn to often for pain relief. My husband is also a type 2 diabetic, and one side effect of the medication he takes is increased cholesterol. We add lemongrass to his homemade essential oil capsules at night because it's recommended for both conditions. For our family, lemongrass makes the list of oils we consider to be life changers.

Infused Living

Create a homemade air freshener by adding 10 drops lemongrass to a small spray bottle. Top with distilled water and shake well before use.

MUSCLE RELIEF MASSAGE OIL

8 drops lemongrass

6 drops lavender

6 drops peppermint

4 drops helichrysum

Sweet almond oil

> Add a drop of lemongrass oil to your favorite Asian recipe.

Combine the essential oils with sweet almond or your carrier oil of choice in a 4-oz. bottle with a pump lid. Massage onto sore muscles or use after exercise.

TAKING A BREATHER

5 drops lemongrass

3 drops clary sage

2 drops patchouli

CLEAR AND CLEAN

2 drops lemongrass

2 drops eucalyptus

2 drops peppermint

2 drops rosemary

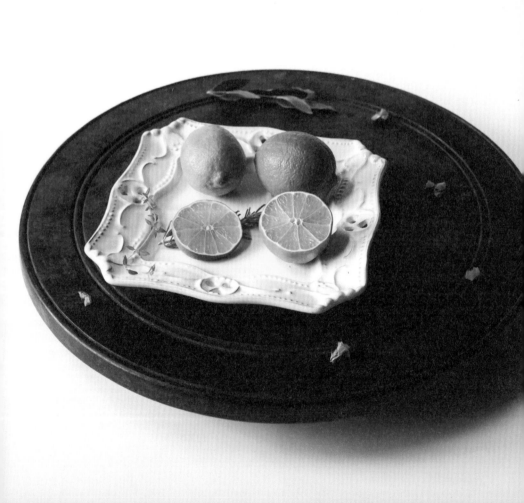

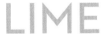

27

LIME

The Essentials: *aromatic, topical, internal, photosensitive*

The refreshing citrus scent of lime conjures thoughts of sun-kissed days and flavorful Mexican cuisine. Start diffusing it to welcome a change of seasons when warmer weather arrives!

Wisdom from the Garden

Lime oil, cold pressed from the rind of the fruit, is known for its bright scent and ability to both lighten the mood and inspire creativity. Lime can be applied to insect bites, support the respiratory system, and improve acne. It possesses antimicrobial, antioxidant,[1] and anti-inflammatory[2] properties. Photosensitivity can occur, so don't apply lime to skin that will be exposed to the sun within the next few hours.

Lime summons the smell of summer in the diffuser and blends well with rosemary, citronella, ylang ylang, jasmine, or lavender along with other citruses such as lemon, orange, grapefruit, or tangerine.

Like Food for Your Mood

Have you ever noticed how a mood can be as contagious as a virus? The state of mind of those around us makes an impact, for better or worse. My cousin called his son a battery charger because of his knack for energizing those around him. On the flip side, have your good spirits ever disintegrated when spending time with someone especially glum? We are social beings, influenced by the attitude of those around us.

Thankfully, essential oils can influence our frame of mind when inhaled. Their small molecules easily pass into the limbic part of the brain, our emotional center. When it comes to essential oils, lime possesses the ability to improve your mood and put a smile on your face, like a favorite playlist coming through your car's speakers. It's a mood booster that teases your taste buds with the flavor of key lime pie and fresh guacamole and evokes thoughts of lazy days at the beach. I love its tart taste in my water and the way lime's sweet scent lasts all day on my diffuser earrings.

Infused Living

Can you brighten someone's mood today? How can you show a friend they have your support and you have their back? Grab a bag of chips, whip up a batch of Fire Roasted Corn Guacamole, add lime oil to the diffuser, and share your time with a friend!

FIRE-ROASTED CORN GUACAMOLE

2 to 3 ears of fresh corn, fire-roasted on a grill or your gas stovetop

5 ripe avocados

3/4 cup pico de gallo

2 to 3 cloves of garlic, minced

¹/₄ tsp. ground cumin

¹/₂ tsp. kosher salt

Fresh cilantro, to taste

2 to 3 drops lime essential oil (start slow and add to taste)

Soak the corn in their husks over-night in water. Shuck and then roast the corn on a grill or the burners of your gas stovetop. Remove the kernels from the cob with a knife and put into a medium bowl. Cut the avocados in half and then use a knife to cut the inside into smaller pieces, which you'll scoop out of the peel and add to the corn. Add the pico de gallo, gar-lic, cumin, salt, cilantro, and lime oil. Stir together and eat with tortilla chips. YUM! Refrigerate leftovers.

Add one or more drops of lime oil to homemade guacamole.

LOVE POTION

3 drops lime

3 drops juniper

2 drops clary sage

SAGE & CITRUS

4 drops clary sage

3 drops lime

2 drops grapefruit

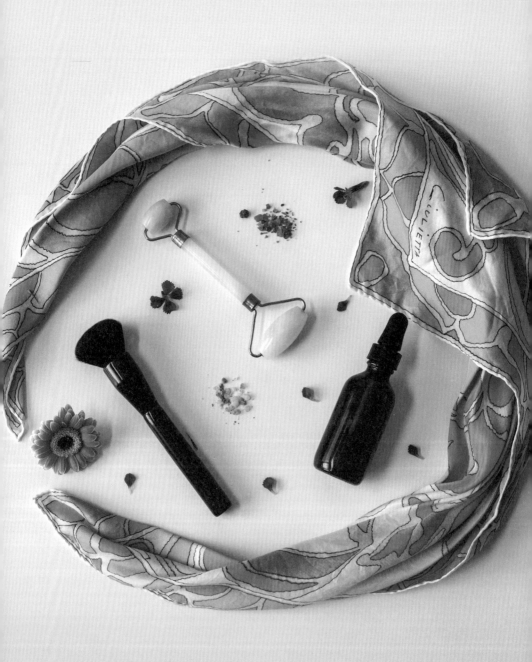

28

MANUKA

The Essentials: *aromatic, topical*

Manuka oil, known for its numerous skin-care benefits, is similar to tea tree but may be even more powerful, with a milder, warmer aroma. This is an oil you want in your collection—a treat for your skin!

Wisdom from the Garden

Manuka oil, steam distilled from the branches and leaves of the manuka plant, is native to New Zealand. It displays antimicrobial activity effective against acne,[1] antibacterial activity effective against the type of bacteria that causes the most staph infections,[2] and "the antimicrobial and anti-inflammatory effects of the oils [are] obtained without adversely affecting the immune system."[3] Traditionally manuka has been used as a sedative, fever reducer, and cough suppressant. It's commonly used to hydrate skin and treat blemishes when added to a facial cleanser or moisturizer, to massage onto a dry or itchy scalp, to support the respiratory system, and to fight nail infections on the feet or hands. Mix a few drops with a carrier oil to make a DIY hair mask.

The sweet, woodsy aroma of manuka blends well with tangerine, orange, bergamot, black spruce, or grapefruit in the diffuser.

Liquid Gold

Our family consumes a lot of honey and agave. For years I've purchased them from wholesale clubs in the biggest sizes available, but a couple of years ago I noticed a new kind of honey—new to me, at least—with a substantially higher price tag. My wholesale club's website currently sells manuka honey, a product of New Zealand, for $99.99 for an 8.8-oz. jar. No, that isn't a typo. It breaks down to $11.36 per ounce. Even at this price, demand outstrips supply. Lawsuits were filed by consumers who discovered the manuka honey they purchased as 100 percent pure was counterfeit (it was actually less than 65 percent manuka honey). *Good Morning America* launched an investigation into the purity of several brands. According to New Zealand's Ministry of Primary Industries, more than five times as much manuka honey is sold worldwide as what their country actually produces.[4] That's not just bad math. It's bad business practiced by companies taking advantage of consumer fervor for this natural wonder.

So what's the big deal? Manuka honey is less in demand for its taste than for its ability to heal wounds and burns, aid digestion, and keep skin smooth. There's even a medicinal grade used topically in hospitals and wound-care clinics. Manuka oil and manuka honey come from the same plant and share similar properties, but some sources say that manuka oil, a highly concentrated essential oil, is much more powerful by weight than the honey. Bacteria keep outsmarting our best antibiotics, but thankfully God, our Intelligent Designer, provided us with plants such as manuka with incredible natural benefits. My son and I incorporate it in our skin-care routines. I appreciate its moisturizing quality, and my son likes the way it improves the condition of teen skin. For its many benefits, powerful manuka oil makes a great addition to your oil arsenal.

Infused Living

Combine 3 drops of manuka oil with ¼ cup Epsom salt in a warm water foot soak and relax while manuka's antifungal properties help keep your feet and toenails healthy.

—

INNER GLOW SKIN SERUM

10 drops frankincense
8 drops cedarwood
8 drops lavender
5 drops manuka
5 drops geranium

Add a few drops of manuka to your facial wash to help clear blemishes.

Combine the oils in a 2-oz. glass bottle
with dropper and top off with grapeseed oil or carrier oil of choice. Shake gently to combine. Apply to face and neck morning and evening.

—

KEEP CALM AND CARRY ON

3 drops manuka
3 drops bergamot
2 drops lavender

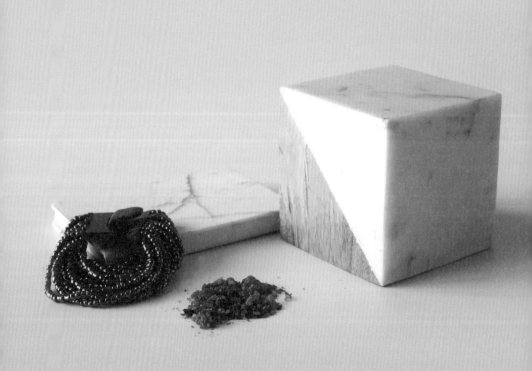

29

MYRRH

The Essentials: *aromatic, topical*

Did you know myrrh is the most popular oil in the Bible? Not only is it mentioned more times than any other aromatic oil, but it was both the first (Genesis 37:25) and the last oil mentioned (along with frankincense) in Revelation 18:13.[1]

Wisdom from the Garden

Rich, earthy-scented myrrh oil derives from steam-distilling the resin of the commiphora tree. Historically, myrrh has been traded and valued in the Middle East and North Africa for thousands of years. It was used for embalming by the ancient Egyptians and as both an anointing oil and painkiller by the ancient Jews. Hippocrates recommended myrrh for sores, and the Romans used it to treat coughs, infections, and worm infestations. Jesus was offered *vinum murratum*—wine with myrrh—at His crucifixion, which would have had an analgesic effect. Myrrh also symbolized death and burial during Jesus's lifetime, and we know gold, frankincense, and myrrh were gifts from the wise men at His birth.

Because of its anti-inflammatory and analgesic properties, myrrh can bring relief from arthritis symptoms.[2] It has antiviral, antibacterial, and antifungal activities[3] and can boost the immune system.[4] Myrrh can kill dormant Lyme disease bacteria, which can cause persisting symptoms after Lyme antibiotic therapy.[5] This thick, moisturizing oil may improve the appearance of chapped skin, wrinkles, and stretch marks, and it has long been used as an ingredient in perfume and incense.

Myrrh's earthy aroma blends well with frankincense, lemon, or lavender in the diffuser.

When You Need Myrrh Focus (bad pun intended)

Because I'm an independent, I-can-handle-it kind of girl, prayer is the most powerful yet underused tool in my kit. Plus I'm easily distracted. (Squirrel!) As soon as I close my eyes, bow my head, and begin to pray, my brain wanders to the most important item on my to-do list, the scheduling conflict I need to resolve, that important text I forgot to send, or the item I keep forgetting to put on the grocery list. It's inevitable. And praying once I get in bed seems to guarantee instant sleep. It's downright embarrassing.

After reading the "Wisdom from the Garden" section about myrrh, you may think there's nothing this oil can't do. That's how I felt while researching it. Some oils synergize well with others, enhancing their effects, and myrrh is also one of those special oils. In addition to its other amazing benefits, the calming, grounding fragrance of myrrh can increase your focus during prayer (I refuse to believe I'm the only one who needs help with this). I just stopped to rub a couple of drops on my face and neck because writing takes concentration too. If you're distractible like me, myrrh may enhance your prayer time. I pray that it does!

Infused Living

Add a few drops of myrrh to your shampoo or conditioner for dry hair or a dry scalp.

EDIE'S FAMOUS FACE SERUM 🥄

1 oz. argan oil
10 drops myrrh
10 drops frankincense
10 drops geranium or patchouli

Fill a 2-oz. glass bottle with a dropper lid halfway full of argan oil and then add the essential oils. Shake gently to combine.

SCAR REDUCING ROLL-ON 🥄

20 drops vitamin E oil
10 drops myrrh
10 drops helichrysum
10 drops frankincense
10 drops lavender
5 drops carrot seed

Add myrrh to skin-care products as a natural moisturizer.

Add the essential oils and vitamin E oil to a 10-ml glass roller bottle and top with sweet almond oil or your carrier oil of choice. Shake gently to combine and before use. Roll onto scar daily.

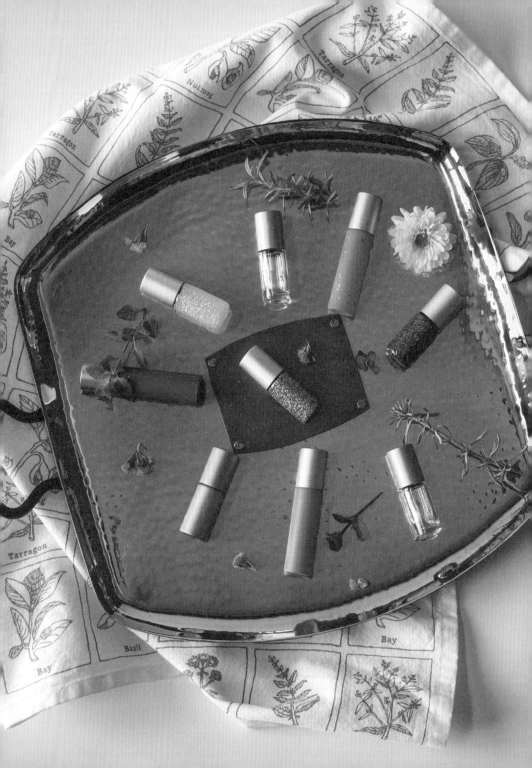

30

MYRTLE

The Essentials: *aromatic, topical, internal*

Myrtle provides powerful support for the endocrine and respiratory systems in an oil mild enough to use with children and the elderly.

Wisdom from the Garden

Myrtle, steam distilled from the evergreen leaves of the large shrub (or small tree), has an extensive history in folk medicine and is mentioned six times in the Bible. Because of its astringent, tonic, and antiseptic characteristics, myrtle has traditionally been used to treat inflammation, chest ailments, hemorrhoids, digestive issues, and skin conditions. Scientific research continues to validate myrtle's long-established uses while exploring its further potential to treat microbial, cardiovascular, gastrointestinal, dermatological, and neurological disease.[1]

Myrtle oil is also known for its thyroid-balancing benefits. In his book *The Chemistry of Essential Oils Made Simple: God's Love Manifest in Molecules*, David Stewart says: "Myrtle oil (Myrtus communis) is an adaptogen that can stimulate an increase or a decrease in thyroid activity depending on a person's condition. Drugs are incapable of such intelligent discriminations and act only in preprogrammed directions, like robots, whether beneficial or not." [2]

The clean, refreshing scent of myrtle blends well with bergamot, lavender, lemon, lemongrass, and spearmint in the diffuser.

Instead of the thorn shall come up the fir tree, and instead of the brier shall come up the myrtle tree: and it shall be to the LORD for a name, for an everlasting sign that shall not be cut off.

Isaiah 55:13

I'm a Believer

It was almost inevitable I would have thyroid problems. When my mother was a teen, her thyroid gland was surgically removed because of a tumor; her mother, my grandmother, had the same surgery. My dad has taken prescription medicine for hypothyroidism for as long as I can remember. At 26 years old, my third pregnancy resulted in a miscarriage, later attributed to undiagnosed hypothyroidism. My second son was 14 months old at the time. Pregnancy can influence thyroid hormone levels, and mine must have bottomed out after I delivered him.

After my diagnosis, it was easy to look back and see the signs. I couldn't make it through the day without a nap, and then I had trouble waking up. Once my thyroid levels were regulated with prescription medication, I functioned normally and my menstrual periods fit the standard 28-day pattern for the first time.

I reconciled myself to taking that little pill every morning for the rest of my life. I knew essential oils could relieve stress, pain, and improve mood, but could they help heal my body from the inside? Based on research and the advice of a friend, I began a taking 4 to 5 drops of an oil blend containing myrtle in my nightly vegetable capsule of essential oils while continuing to take my prescription every morning. Three months later, after reading my bloodwork, my doctor said I could discontinue the thyroid medication I'd taken for 26 years—exactly half my life.

I continue to take oils internally at night. Different people respond differently to different oils, and results may vary. I hoped my dosage of prescription medication would decrease, but I honestly didn't expect to no longer need it. Essential oils have fostered positive change in my body, my health, and my life. I'm a believer.

Infused Living

For thyroid support, apply a drop of myrtle topically over your thyroid gland. To support your endocrine system and adrenal glands, rub it on your lower back just below the ribcage. Apply neat (undiluted) or mix it with a small amount of carrier oil.

BREATHE EASY COUGH REDUCING ROLL-ON

4 drops myrtle
4 drops eucalyptus
4 drops peppermint
4 drops pine

Combine the essential oils in a 10-ml roller bottle and top with your carrier oil of choice. Shake gently to combine. Roll on chest, back, and bottoms of the feet as needed. You can also blend these oils together—without a carrier oil—in an empty essential oil bottle and use them in your diffuser to ease sinus congestion.

> Mix 2 to 3 drops myrtle with 1 to 2 teaspoons carrier oil (like olive oil) and rub on the chest and back to treat a cough.

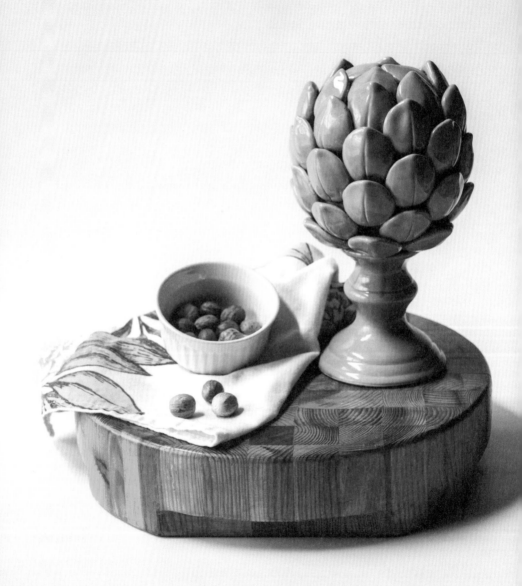

31

NUTMEG

The Essentials: *aromatic, topical, internal*

Nutmeg is not only a culinary oil you might want to have on hand for fall and winter baking, but it also has powerful properties that support your body and energy levels.

Wisdom from the Garden

Sweet and spicy nutmeg oil, steam distilled from the fruit and seeds of the tropical evergreen tree, flavors your food and benefits your body. Traditionally, nutmeg has been used for stomach and kidney disorders, managing rheumatic pain, and healing skin wounds and infections. It exhibits known antioxidant effects;[1] has anti-inflammatory properties;[2] is antibacterial;[3] and may boost mood and libido, benefit heart health, and help control blood sugar.[4] Nutmeg contains compounds that relieve pain, relax blood vessels, lower blood pressure, and benefit the brain. It can help those with Alzheimer's by slowing cognitive decline and promote the recovery of brain tissue following a stroke.[5] Nutmeg supports your body's production of melatonin to help you sleep.

The pungent, spicy aroma of nutmeg blends well with orange, clary sage, eucalyptus, cinnamon bark, clove, or ginger in the diffuser.

Supporting Your Adrenals with Nutmeg

Although adrenal fatigue isn't a named medical condition, undoubtedly sometimes people will experience a collection of nonspecific symptoms— body aches, fatigue, nervousness, sleep disturbances, digestive problems, a craving for salty foods—that may indicate a mild form of adrenal insufficiency, a condition caused by chronic stress. Our bodies release hormones that prepare us to act when faced with the danger of fight-or-flight circumstances, but living in a constant state of stress may cause your adrenal glands to function below the level necessary for you to feel good on a day-to-day basis.

When our adrenal glands are fatigued, essential oils like nutmeg provide effective support by crossing the blood-brain barrier and absorbing into our bloodstream and tissues within seconds, helping to improve our emotional state. They create a hostile environment for things that endanger our cells, such as bacteria and viruses. Because essential oils are so concentrated, they are many times more therapeutically potent than the herbs or plants from which they are derived.

Nutmeg enhances the taste of baked goods; savory recipes; starchy vegetables such as sweet potatoes, squash, and pumpkin; and hot beverages such as hot chocolate, apple cider, and chai tea. Essential oils are potent, so you may only need a drop. Incorporating nutmeg into your diet is a great way to receive the many benefits of this powerhouse oil.

Infused Living

Add 1 or two drops nutmeg oil to a vegetable capsule, a smoothie, under your tongue, or on the inside of your cheek for immune and adrenal support and when you need extra energy.

QUICK SPICY CIDER

2 cups fresh apple cider

1 cup orange juice

3 drops lemon

1 drop nutmeg

1 drop clove

1 drop cinnamon bark

Combine all ingredients in a pot on the stovetop and simmer for 10 minutes until steaming. Serve and enjoy!

Add a drop of nutmeg oil to a glass of eggnog to enhance this holiday treat.

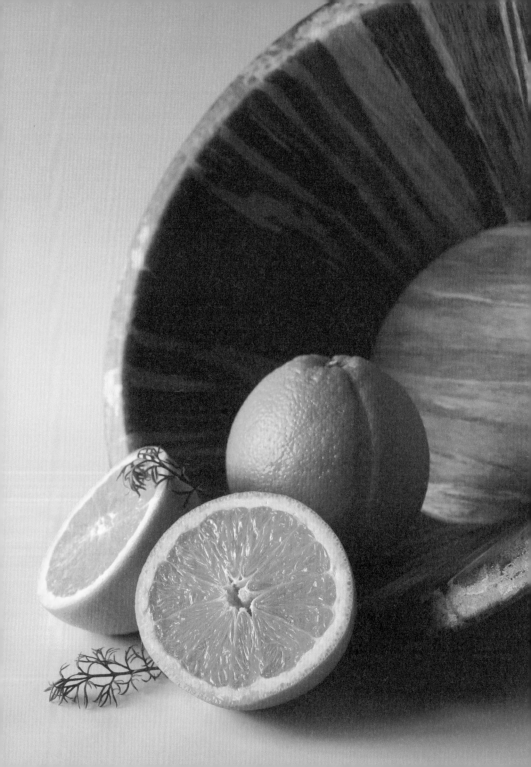

32

ORANGE

The Essentials: *aromatic, topical, internal, photosensitive*

Orange oil is one of my absolute favorites—it's like sunshine in a bottle! It can brighten your mood, calm and relax you, spark creativity, and taste yummy in water. (We diffuse it combined with either lavender, cedarwood, copaiba, or vetiver in our bedroom most nights.)

Wisdom from the Garden

We all know about the benefits of vitamin C from orange juice, but orange oil, cold pressed from the rind of the fruit, has benefits of its own. Orange oil can reduce the appearance of blemishes and improve your complexion when added to your moisturizer or applied blended with a carrier oil such as coconut or grapeseed. The relaxing aroma of orange oil can help ease anxiety, stress, or depression. Its scent can brighten any room and creates a fun and playful environment. Orange oil is also known as a natural aphrodisiac. Search a medical research site like pubmed.gov, and you'll find fascinating studies on the use of orange oil as well as other essential oils.

The sweet, fruity scent of orange combines well with cinnamon bark, grapefruit, or patchouli in the diffuser.

Liquid Sunshine

In college I majored in Russian, but other than a brief stint of tutoring many years ago and teaching one of my sons for his high school foreign language requirement, I haven't done much with it. Honestly, I was more caught up in the challenge than the practical application. I interviewed with a clandestine branch of the government, so I'll have an exciting story for my grandkids, plus occasionally I enjoy reviving my rusty Russian skills by playing with the Duolingo app.

While in college I bought a book called *A Day in the Life of the Soviet Union*. Because I minored in Soviet Studies (another practical choice), I pored through its pages, fascinated by this place and its people I studied daily from a distance. I particularly remember an image of children standing, eyes protected but skin exposed, while receiving light therapy. Parts of Russia (no longer called the Soviet Union, which ceased to exist in 1991) receive very little daylight for extended periods of time. Some areas receive no sunlight for up to two months in winter! The children in the photo were exposed to special lamps believed to help prevent vitamin D deficiency.

The photo sparked a lot of thought. How would I handle the absence of sunlight for days, weeks, or even months on end? Not very well, I think. I walk around the house and open blinds first thing each morning, craving outside light even on the cloudiest day.

Yesterday in the middle of an exceptionally cold and rainy winter, we had a 70-plus-degree day in early February. What did I do? I put orange oil in the diffuser and celebrated an early glimpse of spring. That's one of the beauties of orange essential oil—it can give you a sunshiny-day feeling any time of year!

Infused Living

Need a little sunshine in your day? Add orange oil to hot cider or fruit smoothies for added flavor and health benefits, or wear it on diffuser jewelry to lift your mood. I put a drop on my toothbrush along with toothpaste when I brush my teeth for its delightful flavor!

DIY ROOM REFRESHER

2 drops orange
2 drops grapefruit
2 drops peppermint
2 drops lemon
2 drops bergamot

Combine the oils in a 2-oz. glass spray bottle and top with distilled water. Shake and spray to clear the air! (Always use a glass bottle for recipes with lemon essential oil, which will break down plastic.)

CITRUS KICK!

Mix together 2 drops orange and 1 T. of a natural sweetener to add a kick of citrus to a fruit smoothie, frozen yogurt, or pancake batter.

> Orange oil is photosensitive, so avoid direct sunlight for up to 12 hours on skin where you've applied it.

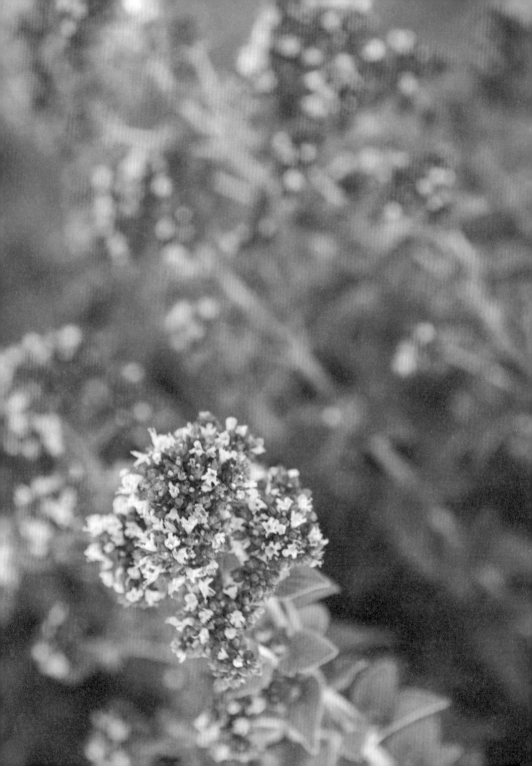

33

OREGANO

The Essentials: *aromatic, topical, internal, hot*

Oregano oil imparts all the health benefits of the fresh herb in an easy-to-store oil, ready whenever you are. Because essential oils are extremely concentrated, you only need a tiny amount—maybe a drop—to enhance your favorite recipes.

Wisdom from the Garden

Oregano oil, steam distilled from the leaves of the plant, has been called nature's antibiotic for its impressive immune system boosting properties. The Greek physician Hippocrates, known as the father of medicine, used it for stomach ailments and as an antiseptic. The twelfth-century German Benedictine abbess Hildegard of Bingen believed food was medicine and therefore the kitchen was a pharmacy. She included oregano in her book *Medicine*.

Oregano has proven effective against multiple common forms of bacteria.[1] Thymol, a major constituent of oregano, has been shown to have antiseptic, anti-inflammatory, antioxidant, and antifungal properties.[2] Oregano has been used for respiratory tract disorders and digestive problems and for skin conditions, including dandruff.[3] It can be used on warts, but beware. Oregano may irritate your skin as well as your wart.

Strong, herbaceous oregano blends well with geranium, lemongrass, or rosemary in the diffuser.

Holding On to Our Health

When I was young, I was fit and active and took my health for granted. Eight pregnancies and deliveries cemented the notion I was practically invincible. Having a baby is exhausting, but when you think about what you accomplished—growing a human being and bringing it forth into the world—it can make you feel like Wonder Woman. Seriously. And while most of my friends have had some silvery strands for years, my daughter-in-law, who is also my stylist, found my first two gray hairs recently while coloring my hair.

The absence of gray and my continued good health confirmed the belief that I'm aging well. Occasionally, however, life shows me I'm not getting any younger and holding on to my health takes intention plus work. Oregano has a long, rich history as a natural form of medicine. My husband and I rotate it among the oils we add to our nightly capsules because it boosts the immune system and cleanses the digestive tract, and I've learned in recent years the importance of guarding our gut health. Blend a drop or two of oregano with a carrier oil and rub it on the bottom of your or your children's feet to help you stay well this winter. Aromatically, oregano creates a feeling of security. I use oils to the best of my ability to care for my family, to keep them secure. God gave them to us for that purpose, and He promises us security in Him too.

If God be for us, who can be against us?

Romans 8:31

Infused Living

Add 1 or 2 drops oregano oil and a carrier oil to an empty vegetable capsule and consume as a dietary supplement to boost your immunity or cleanse your digestive system. Oregano is a hot oil and can irritate your skin, which is why I suggest using it with a carrier oil. The pores on the bottom of your feet are large, and the skin there is less sensitive than other areas of your body, making the spot perfect for essential oil application.

MEDITERRANEAN MARINADE

¾ cup olive oil

½ cup soy sauce

½ tsp. black pepper

½ tsp. kosher salt

2 cloves garlic, minced

2 drops lemon

1 drop oregano

> Add a drop of oregano for extra flavor in Mexican and Italian dishes.

In a bowl, combine all of the ingredients and pour over steak, chicken, or pork chops. Refrigerate in sealed plastic bag for 1 to 4 hours. Discard after use and cook meat as desired.

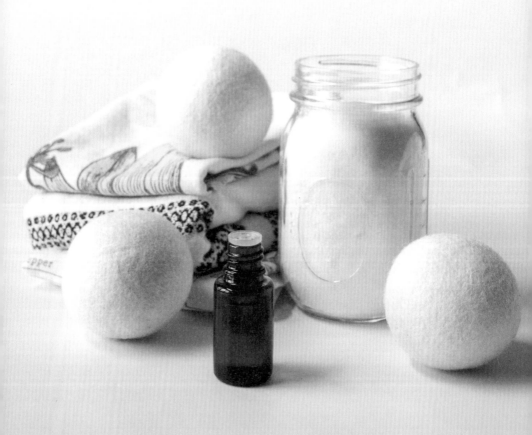

34

PALMAROSA

The Essentials: *aromatic, topical, internal*

Sweet-smelling palmarosa oil is valued in the perfume and cosmetics industry. Geraniol, the primary component of both rose and palmarosa oil, is responsible for their rosy scent. Because it's less expensive to distill palmarosa, which comes from a grass, than rose, which comes from the flower's petals, you'll appreciate palmarosa's lower price!

Wisdom from the Garden

Palmarosa oil, steam distilled from a species of grass native to southern Asia, comes from the same botanical family as citronella and lemongrass. Sometimes called Indian geranium or Turkish geranium, palmarosa is used to flavor food and drinks and to scent perfumes, soaps, and cosmetics. Traditionally used in south Asian communities for support of the digestive, respiratory, and vascular systems, science has confirmed palmarosa's effectiveness in these areas.[1] Physicians in India once prescribed it to lower fever and prevent infection. Palmarosa has antioxidant[2] and anti-inflammatory properties,[3] and has shown broad-spectrum antimicrobial potency.[4] Because palmarosa stimulates new cell growth and speeds healing, it is used to treat not only skin conditions such as eczema and acne but also abscesses and boils. It protects us and our skin by repelling mosquitoes.

Palmarosa blends well with bergamot, geranium, lemongrass, pine, rosemary, ylang ylang, and orange in the diffuser.

How Essential Oils Flood Our Cells

When researching an oil like palmarosa, I'm awed by the things God provides for us in such simple form—a grass—and how perfectly essential oils can distribute a plant's benefits to people who aren't exposed to it in nature. Let me share a bit of chemistry to explain. Our bodies are composed of trillions of cells, more than we can possibly comprehend. An extremely concentrated drop of essential oil contains millions of trillions of molecules—many more than the number of molecules in our bodies. One drop of an essential oil has enough molecules[5] to cover each of our cells with hundreds of thousands of molecules. Here's an example of how that can benefit us: Palmarosa oil was found to be as effective as a commercial insect spray (which, by the way, had a considerable number of potential side effects) at repelling mosquitoes, providing "almost complete protection" against some pretty serious varieties of the insect.[6] Because oils pass through our tissues and straight into our cells, their molecules can spread throughout the body in minutes, no matter where you apply them topically. When you place a drop of palmarosa on your arm, your wrist, or the bottom of your feet, you flood your entire body with its mosquito-repelling properties.[7] The implications are astounding.

Palmarosa oil can soothe the body and the mind. Its sweet, floral fragrance strengthens feelings of security and can be used to help deal with anxiety or grief. Apply it to your wrist or diffuser jewelry and inhale the scent for emotional support when dealing with stress, tension, or nervous exhaustion. Palmarosa moisturizes skin and helps maintain a healthy complexion. It can be added to DIY skin-care products and especially benefits maturing skin. Because of palmarosa's anti-inflammatory properties, use it topically to ease joint pain. Palmarosa is a gift to us, this oil with so many practical applications for our physical and emotional health.

Infused Living

Let fresh, sweet palmarosa brighten your home! Add a few drops to DIY cleaning solutions for floors or countertops. Sprinkle it on wool dryer balls to deodorize your clothes.

> Add equal parts palmarosa and lavender to your diffuser as a sleep blend.

FEMALE HORMONE BALANCING BLEND

5 drops palmarosa
5 drops geranium
5 drops clary sage

Combine the oils in a 15-ml glass essential oil bottle with an orifice reducer cap (the attachment that makes oils drip out instead of pour) and top with coconut oil or carrier oil of choice. Shake gently to combine. Apply a few drops to the back of your neck and forehead to help regulate female hormones.

SPRING HAS SPRUNG

4 drops palmarosa
3 drops bergamot
1 drop cedarwood

FALL DIFFUSER RECIPES

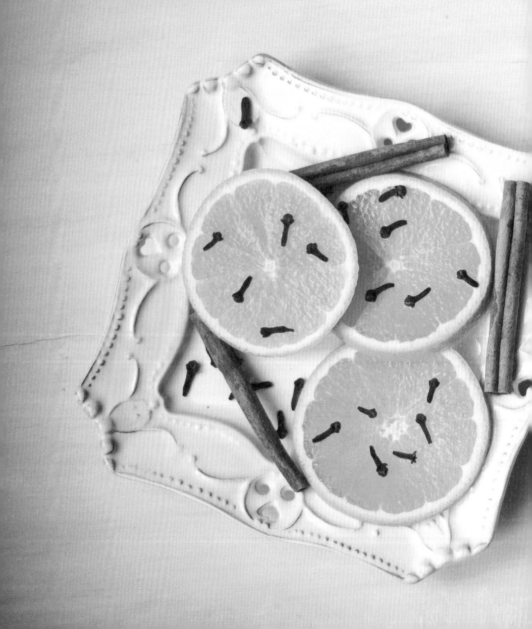

FALL FESTIVAL

3 drops orange

3 drops pine

2 drops cinnamon bark

PUMPKIN PIE

5 drops cinnamon bark

1 drop clove

1 drop nutmeg

A WALK IN THE WOODS

4 drops cypress

2 drops black spruce

2 drops sandalwood

GINGERBREAD COOKIE

3 drops ginger

2 drops clove

2 drops cinnamon bark

1 drop nutmeg

FALLING LEAVES

6 drops orange

1 drop patchouli

1 drop ginger

SNUGGLE UP

3 drops eucalyptus

2 drops juniper

1 drop sage

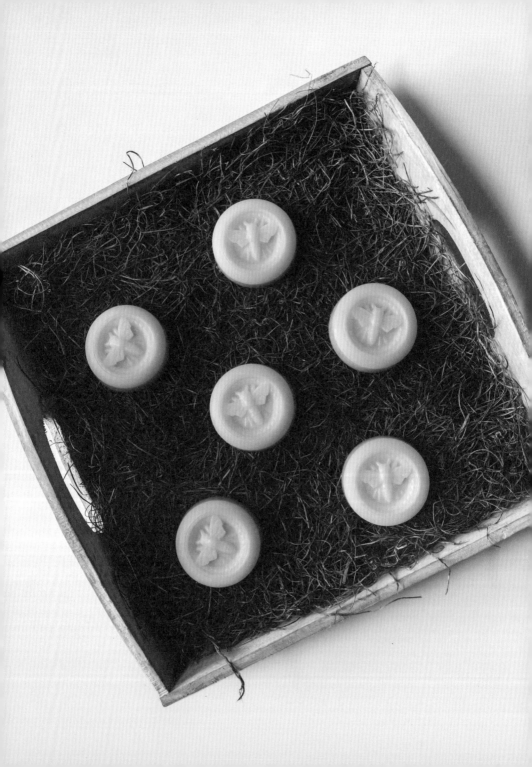

35

PATCHOULI

The Essentials: *topical, aromatic, internal*

If you have a negative connotation with patchouli and think it's a hippie oil, it may be time to take a fresh look at this versatile oil and its benefits. If you're like me, it could become one of your favorites!

Wisdom from the Garden

Patchouli oil is steam distilled from a shrub native to tropical regions in Southeast Asia. It's a thicker oil that can benefit and tone the skin and help prevent wrinkles. Wear its rich fragrance alone or blend it with other oils to create a signature scent. Although patchouli comes from the mint family, it has a musky, sultry smell that has been used to ease stress, anxiety, and depression. While the earthy aroma of patchouli appeals to humans, thankfully, it repels insects.

The aroma of patchouli blends nicely with frankincense, lavender, bergamot, geranium, lemongrass, or cedarwood in the diffuser.

Uniquely, Unmistakably You

Do you ever wish you were more free spirited? Not in a reckless, irresponsible way, but with the innocence and exuberance of youth? Patchouli oil can help you tap into those feelings that make you uniquely, unmistakably you. When you think about patchouli, you might associate it with Woodstock and the 1960s. Its natural scent appealed to hippies and those who favored outdoor living. The sensual, exotic aroma of patchouli can be alluring to both women and men and has a relaxing, grounding effect. Because of the strong associations people have with its smell, the perfume industry doesn't always know what to do with it—whether to incorporate patchouli in a bold or a subtle way.

I often include patchouli in my nighttime routine. I say often because essential oils are more effective when you rotate them periodically, and some produce similar results. They sometimes react differently on people—our bodies may work similarly, but we're each unique. Patchouli combines many of my bedtime needs in one sweet solution: relaxation, hormonal support, emotional balance, skin benefits, and, when I want it, an extra dose of allure. I add a drop to grapeseed oil and spread it over my face and neck, and because it's good for hair, sometimes I rub my fingertips over my scalp with the residue. Try patchouli oil with its unmistakable scent, and you may grow to love it as much as I do.

Infused Living

Experiment with patchouli and complementary oils like orange or lavender to design a personal scent that not only smells amazing but enhances your emotional wellness too.

PERFECT PATCHOULI PERFUME BLEND ⚱

6 drops patchouli

4 drops lemongrass

4 drops orange

4 drops pine

2 drops lavender

2 drops frankincense

> Add patchouli oil to shampoo or conditioner to help control dandruff or an oily scalp.

Combine the oils in a 5-ml glass roller bottle and top with 80 proof vodka or your carrier oil of choice. If you use a carrier oil, use this blend within a year.

DIY LOTION BARS ⚱

½ cup extra-virgin coconut, grapeseed, jojoba, or argan oil

½ cup beeswax pellets

½ cup shea or cocoa butter (or half of each)

10 drops patchouli

10 drops lemon

Silicone molds or muffin tin

Combine the coconut oil, beeswax, and shea or cocoa butter in a pan over low heat or in a double boiler, stirring frequently until the ingredients are completely melted. Add the essential oils and stir until thoroughly combined, and then immediately pour into molds. Let sit overnight before removing the bars from the molds. Store in a cool, dry place. (This recipe can be made with a different complementary pair of oils.)

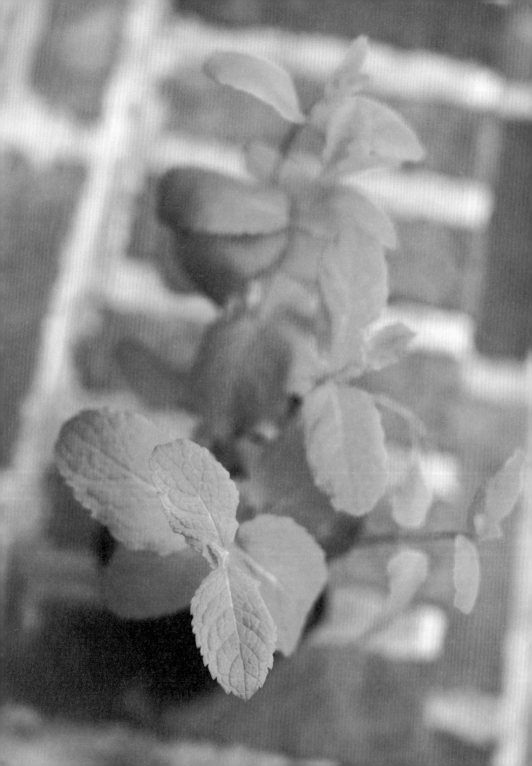

36

PEPPERMINT

The Essentials: *aromatic, topical, internal, hot; avoid for children under two*

Fresh-scented peppermint belongs on any top five essential oils list, along with all-stars such as lavender, frankincense, and lemon. I never leave home without it!

Wisdom from the Garden

Peppermint oil, steam distilled from the leaves and flowering tops of the plant, does so much so well. It improves digestion, boosts energy, invigorates the mind, soothes sore muscles, enhances a glass of water or a recipe, eases nausea and motion sickness, relieves headaches, opens sinuses, provides cooling relief, reduces itching, and helps with topical pain management. Because peppermint is a hot oil, it can cause a hot or warming sensation when applied directly to the skin, so dilute it with a carrier oil for topical application. One of peppermint's greatest superpowers is its effect on insects and other critters. As fabulous as peppermint smells to people, pests such as ants, spiders, cockroaches, mosquitos, and mice hate it, and that's a win for us.

The sweet, invigorating scent of peppermint blends well with lemon, tangerine, lavender, cinnamon bark, rosemary, or sage in the diffuser. Diffuse equal parts lemon, lavender, and peppermint—a.k.a. the Allergy Bomb—to fight seasonal allergies.

Mint Condition

A bottle of peppermint is with me no matter what bag I carry. I may not use it every day, but when I need it, I *need* it. Some seasons are filled with late nights, early mornings, and not enough sleep. When I feel as though I can't stay awake another minute—especially scary while driving!—I pull out the peppermint, hold it under my nose, and breathe deeply until I feel alert again. It's a lifesaver on drowsy days.

I also carry peppermint with me for its ability to kick headaches to the curb. I rub the oil around my hairline or on the back of my neck. Peppermint is a hot oil so I also apply a carrier oil. Sometimes I put a drop under my tongue and leave it there for a minute before swallowing, or I add a drop to my water. If you deal with headaches often, I suggest adding a few drops of peppermint to a 5- or 10-ml roller bottle, topping it off with a carrier oil, and carrying it with you.

The menthol in peppermint oil creates an icy-hot effect when added to a carrier oil for massaging sore muscles. Menopausal women dealing with hot flashes can make a DIY spray by combining a few drops of peppermint with witch hazel in a 4-oz. spray bottle. Spritz your neck, chest, and arms when the heat hits for cooling relief. Inhaling peppermint during a hot flash can help too.

Researchers have found that peppermint oil, taken internally, can improve lung and breathing function and even athletic performance.[1] Since we look for ways to incorporate oils in my son Clayton's cross-country training, he now adds peppermint to his water as an easy way to consume it internally and condition his body for meets.

I diffuse oils in my classroom when I tutor a class of tenth graders one day a week and I often combine peppermint with other oils to keep my students alert. Researchers have determined that peppermint "produced a significant improvement in overall quality of memory."[2] If you smell a scent like peppermint while studying, and then smell it again while being tested, you can recall information more accurately. Diffuser jewelry is an easy way to carry the scent of an oil with you.

Fresh, easily recognizable peppermint is a staple in the collections of both new and experienced oilers, and I know you'll find it necessary to yours too.

Infused Living

Add a few drops of peppermint oil to either homemade brownies or a boxed brownie mix, or add a drop to hot chocolate to create a mint chocolate treat!

___

PEPPERMINT ICE CREAM

2 cups heavy whipping cream
2 cups half-and-half
1 cup sugar
2 tsp. vanilla
½ tsp. sea salt
4 to 6 drops peppermint

> Inhale invigorating peppermint to stay awake and alert in the middle of the day or while driving.

Combine the ingredients, stirring until the sugar dissolves. Freeze according to your ice cream maker's directions.

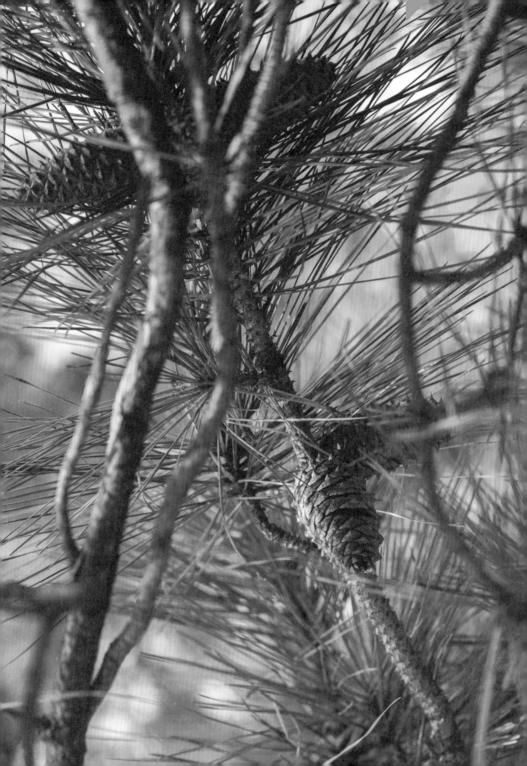

37

PINE

The Essentials: *aromatic, topical*

Because pine is used in so many cleaning products, we associate its scent with clean air and surfaces. Pine oil not only cleans your home but also benefits your body too. It's a fresh-scented, multipurpose oil.

Wisdom from the Garden

Distilled from the needles of the pine tree, pine oil has been used medicinally since the days of ancient Greece and was recommended by Hippocrates. In the past, people stuffed mattresses with pine needles to kill lice and fleas. Today, pine is used to cleanse and deodorize your home and decrease allergies and inflammation in your body. It has known antioxidant and antimicrobial properties[1] and can be combined with a carrier oil to massage sore joints and muscles. Pine supports the respiratory system and has been found to help prevent bone loss.[2]

Eucalyptus and pine are closely related plant species. They can be interchanged in some instances and also work well together by enhancing the action of the other oil. Pine's aroma is both grounding and empowering, relieves stress and mental or emotional fatigue, and can improve your mood.

The fresh, woodsy scent of pine blends well with cedarwood, eucalyptus, lemon, or rosemary in the diffuser.

A Truly Greener Cleaner

It's no wonder the scent of pine fills many commercial products. Pine has long been known for its ability to clean and disinfect. Unfortunately, today most "pine" cleaners contain 3 percent pine oil or less, and sometimes none at all. Manufacturers have replaced the natural cleaning power of pine with synthetic pine fragrance. The scary thing is that commercial cleaners are filled with harmful chemicals. It would be natural to assume the products we purchase to clean our homes would be safe for us and our families, but unfortunately it's a false assumption. On its website, the American Lung Association warns of harmful chemicals contained in household cleaners, even from companies who claim to produce "green" or "natural" products. Greenwashing—the practice of labeling a product as plant-based or natural although it still contains dangerous chemicals—is a misleading but common form of marketing. These products can not only cause eye and throat irritation and headaches, but also contribute to chronic respiratory problems and allergic reactions—and using a combination of different cleaning products creates even more dangerous fumes.[3] You may find all of this as shocking as I did. How did this happen? Because in the United States, manufacturers are not required to disclose all ingredients in their products, and they choose not to police themselves on our behalf.

What can we do? Just say no to household products and cleaners containing "fragrance," an undefined term that can represent a multitude of dangerous synthetic chemicals.[4] Ditch commercial air freshener in favor of pure essential oils in a diffuser. Check your cabinets for products with ingredients that shouldn't be in your home and around your family.

Beware of products with warning labels. If it's dangerous to ingest, should it be absorbed into the clothes on your body or used to clean your dishes? Be an educated consumer and embrace your role as the guardian of your family's health and the one making purchasing decisions.

I don't mean for you to feel overwhelmed. Change can come all at once or in baby steps, but every good choice counts. Don't be surprised if your family doesn't jump on board when you start to purchase different products, especially if they like the ones they have been using. We all resist change. Make pine oil an important part of your family's cleaning routine. Diffuse it to make your home smell as fresh as God's great outdoors!

Infused Living

Make a massage oil from pine plus a carrier oil for sore joints and muscles, and then breathe deeply and relax as you inhale its grounding fragrance.

PINE HARDWOOD FLOOR CLEANER ⚗️

2 cups warm distilled water

¼ cup white vinegar

1 T. olive oil

10 drops pine

10 drops lemon

Combine the ingredients in a 16-oz. glass spray bottle. Sweep floors, spray floor cleaner, and clean with a microfiber mop.

Deodorize your home by diffusing pine oil.

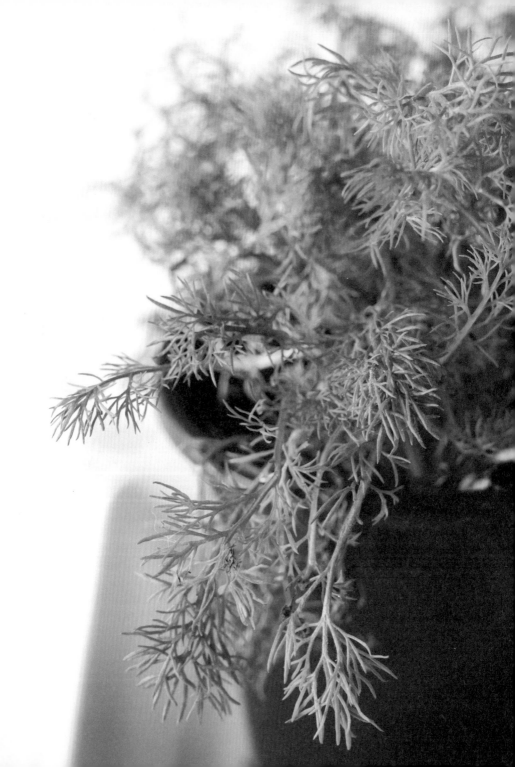

38

ROMAN CHAMOMILE

The Essentials: *aromatic, topical, internal*

Roman chamomile is a delightful oil, capable of soothing skin and calming emotions. I love the relaxing quality of its fresh, fruity aroma.

Wisdom from the Garden

Roman chamomile oil is steam distilled from delicate yellow-and-white wildflowers. Its name translates to "ground apple," reflecting its bright, sweet scent and the low-growing nature of the plant. Historically, it has been used as a natural remedy since ancient times with references found in the medicinal writings of the Egyptians, Greeks, and Romans. What the ancients knew by experience can be proven by modern medicine: Roman chamomile relaxes abdominal cramping,[1] relieves eczema discomfort,[2] and shows antioxidant,[3] antimicrobial,[4] and anti-inflammatory activities.[5] Roman chamomile is used for indigestion, nausea, morning sickness, menstrual cramps, anxiety, sinus and joint pain, skin irritations, and improving sleep, and it's used in cosmetics and perfumes.[6]

The warm, relaxing scent of Roman chamomile blends well with lavender, rose, geranium, or clary sage in the diffuser.

Quality of Life

While researching this oil, I came across a study done with cancer patients that compared the effects of massage with only a carrier oil to a massage with a carrier oil plus Roman chamomile. Researchers found that "the addition of an essential oil seems to enhance the effect of massage and to improve physical and psychological symptoms, as well as overall quality of life."[7] When I thought about that phrase—quality of life—I realized that's exactly what essential oils do for me. They enhance my quality of life. I handle stress better. I sleep better. I've eliminated synthetic toxins from our home and replaced them with oils or oil-infused products. I'm managing menopause, I'm healthy, and I rarely take any prescription or over-the-counter medications.

There are many skeptics when it comes to essential oils, but they don't bother me. I love to witness the "aha!" moments when an oil does something they didn't think it could do and they see God's provision in a whole new way. I've looked for research on humans instead of animals while writing this book, but I've read many of those studies too. It's fascinating how oils affect these creatures because I can't imagine there's a placebo effect. While I knew Roman chamomile reduced anxiety in people, it appears to have an antidepressant effect on rats too.[8] Amazing.

Roman chamomile, as well as the other oils in this book, can improve the quality of our lives in many ways. When you're anxious, open the bottle and breathe deeply. Massage its soothing relief on fatigued muscles. Add 4 or 5 drops to a cup of Epsom salt to create a warm, relaxing bath experience at the end of a long day. Diffuse it to create a peaceful environment for prayer or Bible study. Add it to a carrier oil to moisturize your face. It is my great hope that this book will open your eyes to the wonders of God's creation in new and amazing ways, and that you'll continue to learn how to incorporate oils into your daily life.

Infused Living

For years, mothers have used Roman chamomile to calm children. Apply it to the bottoms of little feet before bed or diffuse it in bedrooms or nurseries for sweet dreams.

CALMING MASSAGE OIL

20 drops Roman chamomile
20 drops ylang ylang
20 drops lavender

Combine the oils in a 2-oz. glass bottle with a pump lid and top with sweet almond oil or other carrier oil of choice. Shake well to combine and before each use. Apply as a calming massage oil.

SLEEPY HEAD

3 drops Roman chamomile
3 drops lavender
3 drops tangerine

Add Roman chamomile to a light carrier oil (grapeseed is a good choice) as a facial moisturizer.

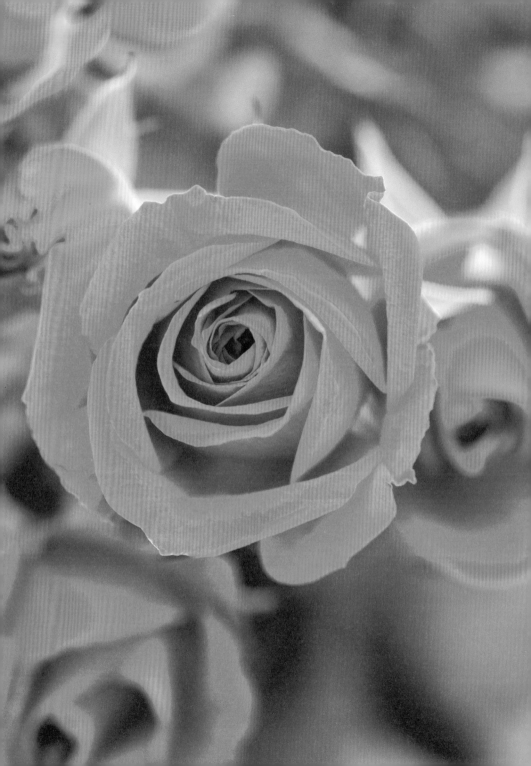

39

ROSE

The Essentials: *topical, aromatic, internal*

It takes 22 pounds of rose petals to produce one 5-ml bottle of high quality rose essential oil—22 pounds! It's one of the most valuable and expensive essential oils you can own, which explains why I hide my bottle out of my children's sight. Rose is an oil I hoard and treasure!

Wisdom from the Garden

Properly distilled rose oil comes from steam distillation of its delicate petals. When applied topically, rose oil has been shown to reduce breathing rates and systolic blood pressure and to bring about feelings of calm and relaxation, making it valuable for relieving stress or depression.[1] Rose oil can benefit dry or aging skin, eczema, bacterial infections, and wounds, and it can reduce inflammation.[2] The intoxicating fragrance of rose serves as a natural aphrodisiac.

Lovely rose oil blends well with jasmine, orange, patchouli, ylang ylang, and bergamot in the diffuser.

Electromagnetic Frequency

Hold on to your hat! We're about to delve into the fabulously fascinating realm of frequency. It might stretch your brain a bit, but don't worry—it does mine too. I remember when my high school physics teacher explained that atoms (of which all things are composed) vibrate even in solid objects, and that if two objects sat against each other for an infinite amount of time, at some point they would begin to merge because of the movement of their atoms. It blew my 17-year-old mind then and still blows my 50-something-year-old mind today. If the atoms of solid objects vibrate, it's not surprising that atoms of living and liquid objects vibrate too.

Essential oils carry electrical charges, which are both healing and healthful. Not only essential oils, but all living things have electromagnetic frequencies that vary from person to person and body system to body system. A healthy person's frequency is higher than an unhealthy person's, and we are more likely to become ill as our frequency dips. The frequencies of essential oils are the highest of known, natural substances—much higher than other plant-based items such as fresh herbs or produce—and rose oil is extremely high among essential oils.[3] Because our body systems operate at different vibrational frequencies, and frequencies vary among oils, it's beneficial to use a variety of oils to help regulate those frequencies. Ultimately, our bodies try to achieve a state of homeostasis, regulating to a normal range, and essential oils can help us in that process.[4] Even inhaling an oil can elevate our body's frequency.

I've always loved roses. This summer we planted several bushes with fuchsia blooms in our yard, and "Rose" is our youngest daughter's middle name. In high school I wore a popular rose-scented perfume; my husband still remembers it from our dating days. Now, however, I avoid the toxins in commercial perfumes and make my own aromatic blends with essential oils. One of my favorites contains a fragrant mixture of sweet floral oils such as rose and jasmine, plus fresh citruses such as orange and bergamot. It smells better than any perfume I ever owned, and applying it helps rather than harms me. Rose oil, with its elevated frequency, benefits my body and calms my mind while sweetening my scent in the process.

Infused Living

Combine rose with complementary essential oils in a 5- or 10-ml roll-on and top with 80 proof vodka or a carrier oil to create a unique signature scent. You can find 21 fabulous aromatics in Melissa Poepping's book *Essential Parfumerie*.[5] I currently carry a roll-on of "M," which features rose oil, in my purse.

Add rose to your face cream for an indulgent, moisturizing treat.

PREMATURE AGING ROLL-ON

8 drops rose
8 drops ylang ylang

Combine the oils in a 15-ml glass essential oil bottle with an orifice reducer cap (the attachment that makes oils drip out instead of pour) and top with argan oil or other carrier oil of choice. Shake well to combine. Apply a few drops to your fingertips and gently apply to your face to reduce signs of premature aging.

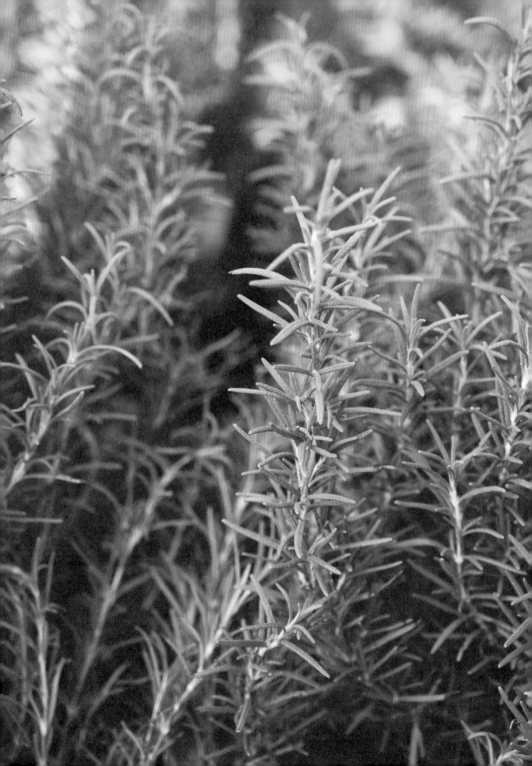

40

ROSEMARY

The Essentials: *aromatic, topical, internal; avoid during pregnancy or if you have epilepsy*

As I write, I'm sitting in a cute little café inhaling the scent of rosemary oil as it drifts up from the homemade macramé feather necklace hanging around my neck. Diffuser jewelry is one of my favorite ways to experience oils!

Wisdom from the Garden

The woodsy aroma of rosemary, steam distilled from a perennial shrub, promotes a sense of clarity. Multiple scientific studies testify that inhaling rosemary oil increases memory function. It also can be a useful tool for learning. Diffuse or inhale rosemary while studying, and then inhale it again when testing or when the need to recall the information arises. Even Shakespeare was aware of this favorable byproduct of rosemary's fragrance.

There's rosemary, that's for remembrance. Pray you, love, remember.

Ophelia, *Hamlet*

Rosemary oil applied to the scalp helps stimulate hair growth, and inhaling it decreases levels of the stress hormone cortisol. Rosemary oil makes a flavorful but potent addition to tomato sauce or as a dip for Italian bread when mixed with olive oil and balsamic vinegar.

Diffusing rosemary can disinfect the air, and its clean, fresh scent blends well with basil, eucalyptus, lavender, peppermint, or pine oil.

The Stuff of Memories

The writing workshop leader gave the following instructions: "Close your eyes and remember a time when you felt completely safe." Soon, the memory surfaced. As a little girl, I sat by my dad in church and extended an arm toward him, palm up, practically begging him to drag his fingertips up and down my arm, wrist to elbow, over and over again. The gentle motion soothed me as a restless child and, as an adult, still recalls to me a feeling of safety and contentment.

I remember how my dad's mom made special treats when we visited: fried potatoes, vanilla malts, and warm chocolate pudding. She cheered loudly at my softball games, although sometimes she yelled, "Three up, three down!" when our team was at bat. My mom's mom was a preacher's wife who served steaming cocoa and homemade chocolate-covered cherries on Christmas Eve and pie plates piled with hot biscuits—butter and sorghum on the side—when I got home from school.

I wonder what mundane moments embed themselves in the hearts and minds of my children. Is it our impromptu trips out for ice-cream sundaes? Will they remember when I read *A Wrinkle in Time* by lamplight in our darkened room, night after night, while they curled under blankets on our bed or snuggled with our dog on the floor? That you can learn all kinds of things if you have an inquisitive mind, a good work ethic, and decent study skills?

I'm new to this grandparent game, but I see that parts of its charm are the chance to revisit fond memories of raising our own children and to watch our grandchildren discover their own favorite things, from foods to books and board games, as the next generation of our family begins its story and I create memories for my children's children.

As a writer, rosemary is one of my favorite oils. It helps me to clear my head and tap into memory, the source of my stories. This life is full of beautiful memories just waiting to be made. It's amazing how much more focused I feel while inhaling rosemary.

Infused Living

Take a favorite food to a friend this week. My friend Melissa loves my snickerdoodles and her mom loves my yeast rolls, so I bake and take them to church lunches to treat them. It makes all of us happy. Wear rosemary oil on diffuser jewelry to improve memory while studying for and then taking a test.

SPA DAY

1 drop rosemary
1 drop ylang ylang
1 drop lavender
1 drop peppermint
1 drop orange
1 drop bergamot

Connect a small USB diffuser to your computer to diffuse rosemary while working on a project.

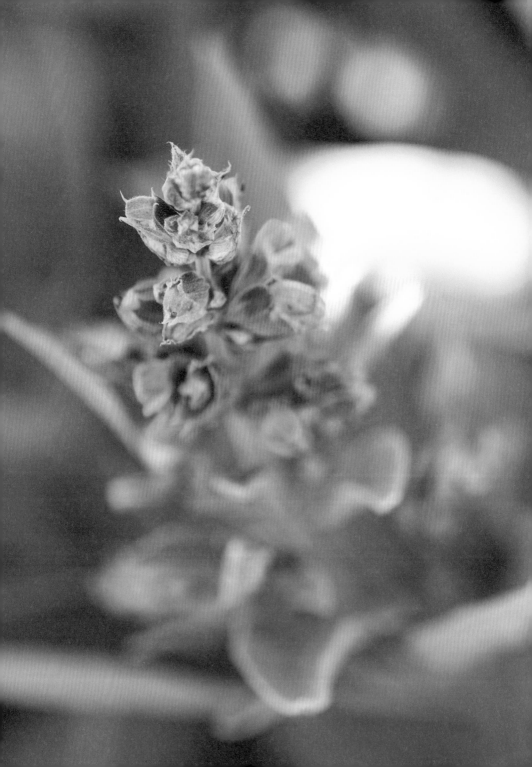

41

SAGE

The Essentials: *aromatic, topical, internal; avoid during pregnancy or if you have epilepsy*

Sage oil, as with the fresh or dried herb, can enliven the flavor of savory dishes in your kitchen. Because oils are potent and concentrated, start with just a drop and add more if desired.

Wisdom from the Garden

The essential oil of sage, a member of the mint family, is distilled from the plant's leaves. Not only can sage, an ancient herb, season meat, poultry, fish, and other savory dishes, but it may benefit us physically as well. Part of its Latin name, *salvia*, comes from the word for salvation. Romans considered sage to have medicinal value and used it, among other things, to stop wounds from bleeding. Historically, sage was used as a fertility drug by the ancient Egyptians. Herbalists have long recommended tea made from sage leaves for sore throats and to dry up a mother's milk once her baby is weaned. They noted its ability to improve memory and sharpen the senses. Today sage tea is called the thinker's tea. Sage has been found to have anti-inflammatory, antiseptic, and antibacterial properties.[1]

It has been used traditionally to treat menopausal symptoms, and one study showed a significant reduction in hot flashes in women who took a daily capsule of fresh sage for eight weeks.[2]

The earthy, herbaceous aroma of sage blends well with bergamot, lavender, lemon, peppermint, or rosemary in the diffuser.

Rediscovering Yesterday's Medicine

Most of the oils in this book come from plants historically considered to have medicinal value. They may have been discovered in King Tut's tomb; used by the Greek physician Hippocrates, who was credited with the phrase, "Let food be thy medicine and medicine be thy food"; mentioned in the writings of Hildegard of Bingen, a German abbess who compiled books on herbal treatments and the human body and saw a connection between medicine and gardening; worn by the ancient Romans, whose physicians received much practical experience on the battlefield; or included in *The Pharmacopeia of the United States of America,* a book containing a list of medicinal drugs, their effects, and directions for use. Many of the recipes recommended by early doctors contained herbs and plants that were found close to their patients' homes and eaten fresh. You could grow your medicine in your garden and then prepare it in your kitchen.

Although ancient cultures—including the Egyptians, Greeks, Romans, and Israelites—prized and used aromatic oils, essential oils regained popularity after World War II because of their desirable fragrances and newly rediscovered capabilities. French physician Dr. Jean Valnet treated injured soldiers with essential oils during World War II and reintroduced natural remedies and their practical application into modern medical research. Today more than 10,000 references to essential oils can be found in the US National Library of Medicine's free, digital database at pubmed.gov as modern research into ancient remedies continues.

Nature only plays a small part in much of modern medicine, although many over-the-counter and prescription medications contain active ingredients derived from plants. As a society, we relinquish control of our health to the doctor and the pharmacist instead of considering our own instincts, the work of the farmer, and the blessings God provides through nature. Information is everywhere, as readily available as a web search from your phone or time invested in a book like this. Become an advocate for your and your family's health. Using culinary oils such as sage combines the benefits of garden-based medicine from the past with the modern convenience of a bottle on your shelf. Sage goes in my and my husband's nightly oil capsules, which have been game-changers for our health. Join us in rediscovering the wisdom of ancient civilizations!

Infused Living

Take sage as a dietary supplement to support your digestive system, either in recipes or empty vegetable capsules designed for internal consumption of essential oils.

—

NATIONAL FOREST

3 drops sage

3 drops pine

2 drops peppermint

1 drop spearmint

Incorporate sage oil into a flavorful Thanksgiving feast!

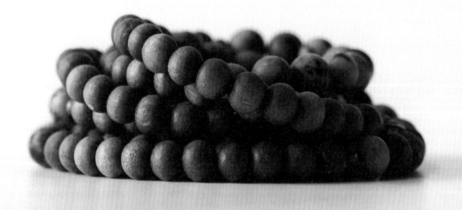

42

SANDALWOOD

The Essentials: *aromatic, topical*

Sandalwood oil, also known as *aloes* in the Bible, appears in both the Old and New Testaments and was one of the burial spices used for the body of Jesus Christ.

Wisdom from the Garden

Steam-distilled from the wood of the aromatic tropical tree, sandalwood is one of the world's oldest forms of incense and remains popular in the perfume and cosmetics industries. The Egyptians used it for embalming the dead. Sandalwood has been used in Indian folk medicine and Chinese traditional medicine for both physical and mental ailments, including urinary tract infections, digestive problems, anxiety, fatigue, fever, the common cold, sore throats, mental disorders, insomnia, high blood pressure, and low libido. Today's research shows that sandalwood reduces anxiety,[1] promotes skin cell growth and wound healing,[2] possesses antimicrobial,[3] anti-inflammatory, and antioxidant properties, and has been used to successfully treat acne, psoriasis, eczema, and common warts.[4]

The sweet, woodsy scent of sandalwood oil blends well with cypress, lemon, myrrh, spruce, frankincense, ylang ylang, lime, orange, patchouli, and lavender in the diffuser.

Of Great Value

Sandalwood, one of the world's most expensive oils, comes from one of the world's most expensive trees. Unlike most aromatic wood, sandalwood retains its fragrance for years, even decades. As the tree slowly grows, essential oil develops in the roots and heartwood, the dense inner part of the tree trunk that yields the hardest timber. The oil is of higher quantity and quality in mature trees between 40 to 80 years old. It's at the end of the tree's natural life when it contains the greatest volume, meaning sandalwood oil can be responsibly harvested from dead or dying trees.

After the death of Christ, Nicodemus and Joseph of Arimathea used oils of myrrh and sandalwood to prepare His body for burial. The quantity of oils used would be valued at more than $150,000 today. This private act of love shows us not only that these men were quite wealthy, but also how deeply they regarded and revered their Lord.[5]

I occasionally come across research that shows the potency of oils and then ends with a recommendation to try to recreate their properties in synthetic form. Just because oils weren't created in a laboratory, it doesn't mean they aren't effective. They were perfectly formed by the greatest scientist of all time, God Himself. As David Stewart so eloquently explains, a drug's weakness is an oil's strength:

> The endless and unpredictable variation in the composition of a particular species of oil that is considered so undesirable and disadvantageous to druggists and doctors is, in fact, one of the most desirable and advantageous qualities of an essential oil. Because of their variability and unpredictability, bacteria can never anticipate ways to resist an

essential oil. Therefore, resistance to essential oils can never develop. Oils that were effective against bacteria in Egypt and Israel thousands of years ago are just as effective today as they ever were. Their effectiveness will never diminish even thousands of years hence.[6]

Sandalwood oil, highly valued in biblical times, is equally precious today. I'm grateful the gifts of plant species throughout the world are available to us because of modern distillation and distribution methods.

Infused Living

Add a few drops of sandalwood to your daily moisturizer to reduce blemishes and experience its incredible benefits for the skin. Inhale at bedtime to calm your mind and enhance deep sleep.

———

HEALING BODY BUTTER ⚱

³⁄₄ cup shea or cocoa butter
¹⁄₄ cup sweet almond oil
¹⁄₄ cup grapeseed, sunflower, or coconut oil
¹⁄₄ cup vitamin E oil
15 drops sandalwood
10 drops frankincense
5 drops cypress
5 drops lavender
5 drops patchouli
5 drops ylang ylang

Diffuse sandalwood for focus, clarity, and to make your house smell like a spa!

Melt the shea or cocoa butter in a pan over low heat. Remove from heat, cool slightly, and then stir in the carrier oils and essential oils. Place in refrigerator or freezer to chill until partially solidified, and then whip until mixture forms a butterlike consistency. Store in 16-oz. Mason jar.

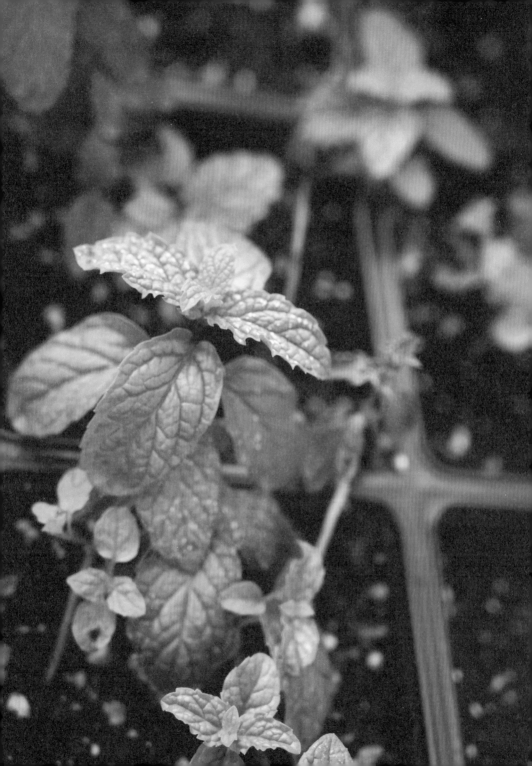

43

SPEARMINT

The Essentials: *topical, aromatic, internal*

Rather than chewing gum, try spearmint essential oil when you need extra refreshment. Spearmint is softer and milder than peppermint, with a fresh, minty taste and an invigorating scent.

Wisdom from the Garden

Spearmint oil, steam distilled from the leaves of the plant, increases your metabolism and supports good digestive health. Add 1 or 2 drops to water or rub the oil directly on your tummy; it's not hot on the skin like peppermint. Spearmint oil can provide relief for itchy or irritated skin and help reduce anxiety. Its sweet flavor can be added to recipes. Remember, though, that less is more because essential oils are highly concentrated.

Minty spearmint mixes nicely with basil, lavender, peppermint, or rosemary in the diffuser.

The Importance of Reaction

Our bodies can have a fascinating response to essential oils. Author Jen O'Sullivan says if you have an extreme reaction to an oil—you hate it or you almost crave it—then your body needs it.[1] The first time I added spearmint to my water, I disliked it so much I poured it out. It's the only time I've added an oil to my water and didn't drink it. A few months later a friend talked about how much she loved spearmint in her water and I was stunned. I assumed everyone thought it tasted as bad as I did. I tried it again and had the complete opposite reaction. I carried it in my purse for a few weeks because I wanted it available at all times.

These contradictory reactions puzzled me until a few months ago when I started using an oil blend in an intentional and specific way to deal with a health problem I've had more than half my life. The blend's primary ingredient is spearmint, and the results were astounding with a clear conclusion. My body needed spearmint all along, both when I was repulsed by it and when I craved it. If I'd understood that the intensity of my reaction meant something, I would have paid more attention to it at the time.

If you experience a strong negative or positive response to an essential oil, research its possible applications to discover why you may need it. An essential oils reference guide in book or app form can be a big help.

Infused Living

When you suffer from stomach discomfort, add a drop of spearmint oil to water or tea to calm your tummy and improve digestion.

———

DIY MOUTHWASH 🪔

2 cups distilled water

5 drops spearmint

3 drops peppermint

2 drops orange

1 drop tea tree

Combine the ingredients in a 16-oz. Mason jar with a lid and shake well. Use as mouthwash after brushing.

MIND AND MOOD EUCALYPTUS SPEARMINT SUGAR SCRUB

¾ cup sugar
¼ cup grapeseed, coconut, or jojoba oil
5 drops spearmint
5 drops eucalyptus

Combine the ingredients in either one 8-oz. or two 4-oz. Mason jars.

Pamper your hands and body with the combination of sugar's ability to exfoliate, the spa day vibe of spearmint and eucalyptus essential oils, and the skin softening power of grapeseed oil. You won't believe how soft your skin will feel!

Add more carrier oil (the fatty vegetable oil, not the essential oil) if needed to reach your preferred consistency. A cute spoon is fun for scooping out the sugar scrub. Look for them at your local thrift store.

LAKE DAY

3 drops cypress
3 drops lavender
2 drops tangerine
2 drops spearmint

Diffuse spearmint and peppermint together for a minty pick-me-up blend.

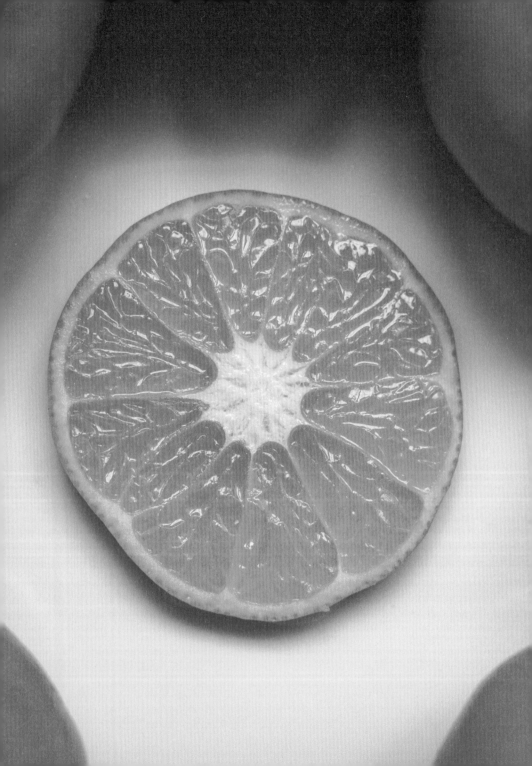

44

TANGERINE

The Essentials: *topical, aromatic, internal, photosensitive*

Tart, tangy, and terrific, tangerine oil brings a burst of citrus freshness to your water, recipes, or the air via your diffuser. It's like orange oil with an extra kick!

Wisdom from the Garden

The refreshing, citrusy fragrance of tangerine appeals to both adults and children. Its happy scent can boost your mood. Essential oils are different than fruit juices. Tangerine oil is cold pressed from the rind of the fruit. Tangerine, as well as other citrus oils, has been shown to have antioxidant, anti-inflammatory, antimicrobial, and antiallergy activities.[1] Add tangerine to your facial cleanser for fresh, beautiful skin or inhale it for a positive attitude adjustment.

Fruity, calming tangerine blends well with bergamot, clary sage, frankincense, geranium, grapefruit, lavender, or lemon in the diffuser.

Olfactory Optimism

Have you ever noticed that optimism is influenced by our mindset more than our circumstances? We all know people who have very little from a worldly point-of-view but live joyful lives, while others who appear to have it all are depressed or miserable. Clearly joy comes from within more than without. If we allow our relationships and the circumstances of our lives to define our outlooks, it doesn't take much to knock us down. The world can always do that. When we focus on God and our worth in Him, He fills the places in our hearts that the world never will. We can learn a lot about contentment from these words by the apostle Paul:

I have learned in whatever state I am, to be content: I know how to be abased, and I know how to abound. Everywhere and in all things I have learned both to be full and to be hungry, both to abound and to suffer need. I can do all things through Christ who strengthens me.

Philippians 4:11-13 NKJV

We don't need to rely on the world for our joy. We have God within us and the good gifts He gave us, including essential oils, at our disposal. Seek peace in Him and let tangerine's sunny scent boost your mood, calm your mind, and restore your optimism.

Infused Living

Incorporate tangerine in your kitchen by adding it to marinades, salad dressings, baked breads, and desserts, or to take the taste of your water up a notch and encourage you to drink more.

HOLIDAY WASSAIL 🥣

6 cups fresh apple cider

2 cups pineapple juice

5 drops tangerine

5 drops clove

5 drops cinnamon bark

Combine the ingredients in a pan on the stovetop and heat at medium-high until hot, or add ingredients to a slow cooker and heat slowly throughout the day. Keep covered or add additional oils before serving because heating for a long time or uncovered is like diffusing the oils into the air.

SWEET FRUIT SMOOTHIE 🥣

1½ cups frozen strawberries, mangoes, peaches, blueberries, or pineapple

12 oz. cold water or almond milk

3 drops tangerine

Add all ingredients to a blender and mix until smooth. Drink immediately.

Rub a drop of tangerine between your hands and inhale some airborne optimism.

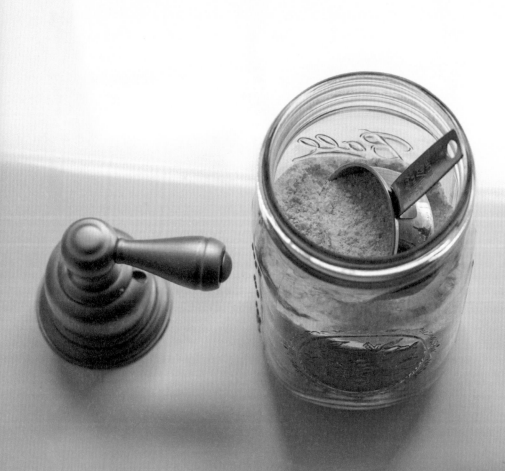

45

TEA TREE

The Essentials: *aromatic, topical*

It's no wonder tea tree, also known as *Melaleuca alternifolia,* is one of the most well-known essential oils. Because it's both cleansing and refreshing, many skin-care and cleaning products include tea tree oil.

Wisdom from the Garden

Even if you're new to essential oils, you've probably heard of multipurpose tea tree oil. When Captain James Cook sailed around the world in the 1700s, he brewed tea from the leaves of Australia's *Melaleuca alternifolia* tree, giving it a new nickname: the tea tree. Aboriginal Australians have long understood the healing powers of tea tree, and the oil was included in Australian soldiers' kits as an antiseptic during World War II. Distilled from the leaves of this tree, tea tree oil is used for acne, dandruff, insect bites, and wound care, and it has been tested for its anti-inflammatory, antibacterial, and antiviral properties.[1] Add a couple drops to water and swish in your mouth for a homemade mouthwash[2] or add a few drops to your shampoo to combat dandruff.

Use tea tree as a natural deodorizer in DIY room sprays. The medicinal, spicy aroma of tea tree blends well with lavender, rosemary, or citrus oils in the diffuser.

Become a DIY Ninja with Tea Tree Oil

I used to jokingly/not so jokingly ask my mom how old you had to be in our family to not battle blemishes on your face. She had no good answer because no end seems to be in sight. I'm in my fifties and still deal with them occasionally (writing this chapter seemed to summon two new ones). Whenever it happens, tea tree is one of my go-to oils. I dab a drop on the offending spot and, in no time, it's gone! My teen son uses it regularly on his face too. Tea tree is a powerful oil and can cause contact sensitivity for some people, but you can dilute it by adding a mild carrier oil, such as grapeseed or coconut, or by applying it with fingers dampened with water.

The research required to write this book has taught me so much. I would read about an unfamiliar way to use a familiar oil and then head straight to my stash to try it, which led me to make a tea tree mouthwash for the first time today. Now I will include tea tree among my choices of oils to add to my toothpaste at night.

One of the benefits of keeping an ever-expanding variety of essential oils on hand is the ability to eliminate chemical-laden air fresheners from our home, instead customizing health and beauty products with the oils we love and need. Diffusing a few drops of tea tree, alone or combined with lemongrass or another fresh citrus oil, helps eliminate household odors while imparting health benefits, unlike toxic commercial air fresheners which contain allergens, hormone disruptors, and worse.[3] A wide variety of health and beauty products contain tea tree oil, including shampoo, conditioner, skin and scalp treatment, and deodorant. Add a few drops of tea tree oil and amp up your favorite products!

Infused Living

Mix tea tree oil with a carrier like vitamin E oil and massage into dry or cracked cuticles to moisturize and fight infection.

BREAKOUT BUSTER ROLL-ON 🍶

8 drops tea tree

8 drops palmarosa

6 drops copaiba

6 drops lavender

4 drops manuka

Combine the oils in a 10-ml glass roller bottle and top with grapeseed oil. Shake gently to combine and before each use. Roll onto problem skin areas to control breakouts.

DIY OATMEAL BATH SOAK 🍶

1 cup quick oats

1 cup Epsom salt

½ cup baking soda

15 drops lavender

10 drops tea tree

5 drops frankincense

Add a few drops of tea tree oil to wool dryer balls for fresher clothes.

Grind the oats in a food processor or blender until they have a fine, flour-like texture. Then thoroughly mix all the ingredients and store in a glass jar. Add one cup to your bathwater for a sweet-smelling, skin-soothing treat!

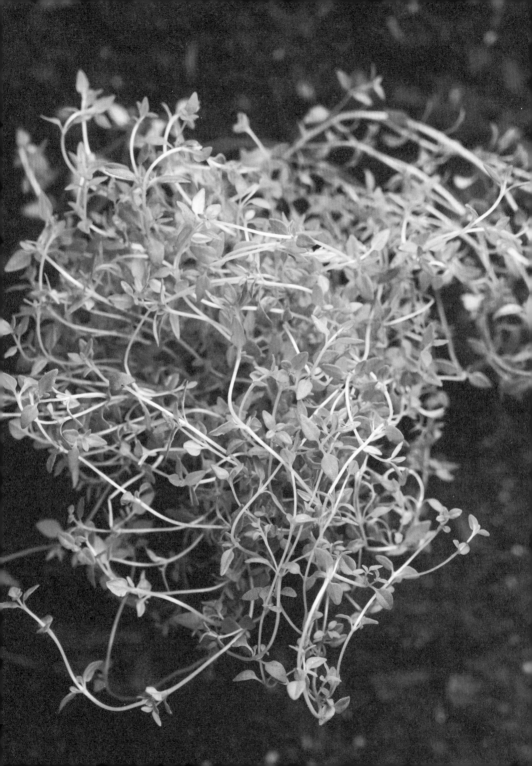

46

THYME

The Essentials: *aromatic, topical, internal, hot*

If you're looking for an oil to support you during winter months, add thyme to your personal collection. This common garden herb offers many benefits!

Wisdom from the Garden

Steam-distilled from the leaves of the plant, thyme oil has a rich and fascinating history. The ancient Egyptians used it for embalming. The Romans believed it was an antidote for poison and an aid in battle, symbolizing courage and honor. Medieval knights carried the herb, a gift from their ladies, into battle and when they traveled. Thyme was listed in a European reference book (dated AD 78) for herbal remedies and also in *Medicine,* written by the Benedictine herbalist Hildegard of Bingen (1098–1179). When used for cooking, thyme can help protect against food spoilage. Today thyme oil is known for its antiaging and immune-boosting properties.

Combine the strong, hot aroma of thyme with oregano, clove, or eucalyptus in the diffuser to support the respiratory and immune systems, or with lavender, lemon, and peppermint to freshen the air and relieve physical and mental fatigue.

———

Whereby no tattered herbage tells
Which way the season flies,
Only our close-bit thyme that smells
Like dawn in Paradise.
Rudyard Kipling, "Sussex"

———

A Line of Defense

I have a friend who kindly offered me the use of her vacation home to get away and work on this book. What a gift! A few days before leaving, I developed an infection around one eye, possibly caused by an insect bite, that required a trip to the doctor and two antibiotics in case it could be staph. When the doctor says, "This is really close to your brain," and "This could lead to meningitis," you pay attention. I Googled meningitis, and ain't nobody got time for that!

(This is a good time to mention that essential oils can sometimes keep you away from the doctor's office, but be smart and know when you need to visit. Modern medicine has its place.)

So here I sit, warm compress on my eye, writing in a house with an idyllic view: large pasture, grazing cows, red-roofed barn, white-steepled church in the distance, surrounded by the Great Smoky Mountains. I'm following the doctor's orders but also taking steps of my own. Antibiotics can destroy gut health because they don't differentiate between good and bad bacteria; they attack it all. The proper balance of bacteria in my gut is crucial to overall health, not only for my digestive system but my immune system and hormone production too. When the good bacteria are killed off, it allows other organisms, such as yeast, to multiply. I'm loading up on probiotics, including Greek yogurt, dairy and dairy-free yogurt drinks, and kefir, all of which stimulate the growth of good intestinal bacteria.

As well as protecting my gut health, I'm also using specific essential oils to help attack the bad bacteria. With time and overuse of antibiotics, some bacteria have become resistant to them. (Google MRSA for more information.) Researchers are discovering the benefits of combining natural and pharmaceutical medicines and that some essential oils, thyme included, can work synergistically with antibiotics.[1] Because probiotics are live organisms, I take them a few hours apart from the antibiotics and essential oils so these medications don't destroy the fragile probiotics along with the bad bacteria. I don't want to eliminate one infection and create another in the process.

I'm thankful to have thyme oil as a powerful and essential part of my wellness arsenal!

Infused Living

Use a thyme oil that has been labeled for internal consumption in place of the dried herb in pasta or poultry dishes.

PERFECT PASTA SAUCE

Take the taste of homemade or jarred pasta sauce up a notch by adding 1 drop each thyme, rosemary, and basil oil.

Dilute in a 1:4 ratio (1 drop thyme with 4 drops carrier oil) and apply to sore muscles.

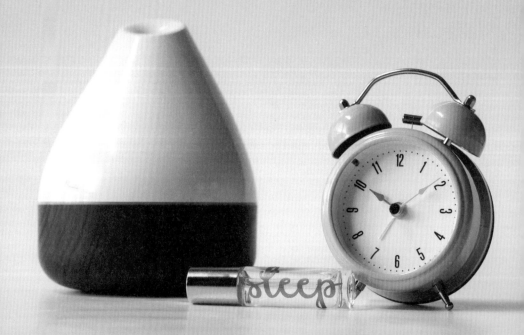

47

VALERIAN

The Essentials: *topical, aromatic, internal*

If you have trouble sleeping, let valerian oil come to your rescue! I prefer taking it internally in vegetable capsules (designed for holding essential oils) because of its smell.

Wisdom from the Garden

Valerian is steam distilled from the root of the plant and has been used medicinally since the time of the ancient Greeks and Romans. Its therapeutic properties were noted by Hippocrates. Nicknamed "nature's Valium," valerian is known for its sedative properties and benefits to those who suffer from insomnia. Valerian may lessen anxiety in stressful situations.[1] Studies show that it can reduce sleep disorders in menopausal women [2] as well as the frequency and severity of hot flashes.[3] Valerian has also proven to lessen physical, emotional, and behavioral symptoms of premenstrual syndrome.[4]

Valerian combines well with cedarwood, lavender, patchouli, or rosemary in the diffuser.

The Oil That Almost Didn't Make the Book

To be honest, valerian smells really bad. Although the plant's flowers are sweet, valerian oil comes from the root, which has a strong, unpleasant odor. When I explained to a friend that I felt obligated to tell you, my readers, that valerian stinks, she asked, "Do you have to include it?" I thought for a minute and then replied, "No, I don't." At that moment I made the executive decision to strike valerian from this book, promptly removed it from my list of 50 oils, and never looked back until recently—after unsuccessfully trying to reset my internal clock after a trip. I'd spent a week in a state two time zones away and couldn't seem to adjust my sleep schedule when I returned home. Research suggested valerian for insomnia and sleep disturbances, so I pulled out my dusty bottle and gave it another try.

I used to diffuse this oil, and because of that, I had remembered its smell more than its effect. After a few days of better sleep, though, I knew valerian had earned its place back on my book's list. And although inhaling a drop in my cupped hands is better than diffusing, I've now determined that internal consumption is best. If you suffer from insomnia, you may discover what people have known for thousands of years: Valerian works.

Infused Living

Put two drops of valerian in a capsule and take in the evening for more restful sleep, or combine a few drops with coconut or another carrier oil in a glass bottle with a roll-on attachment and rub on the bottoms of your feet and big toes at bedtime.

JUST RELAX ROLL-ON

25 drops valerian

25 drops vetiver

25 drops cedarwood

25 drops geranium

Combine the oils in a 15-ml glass roller bottle and fill it to the top with olive or other carrier oil. Roll on wrists, temples, back of the neck, or behind the ears for relaxation.

GOOD NIGHT, SLEEP TIGHT FOOT SOAK

3 drops valerian

5 drops tea tree

1 T. coconut oil or carrier oil of choice

1 tsp. salt

Combine ingredients in warm water. Mix well and soak feet for 15 minutes at bedtime.

SLEEPY TOWN

4 drops valerian

3 drops pine

3 drops orange

Add a few drops of valerian to an Epsom salt foot soak to relax before bedtime.

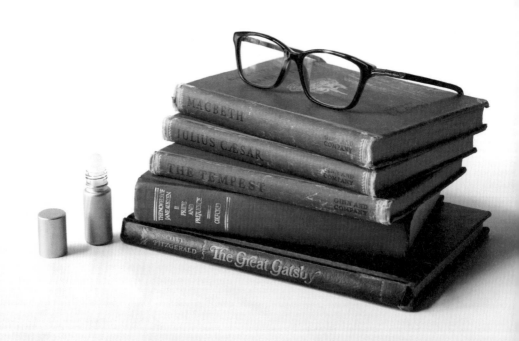

48

VETIVER

The Essentials: *aromatic, topical*

The earthy, exotic, and woodsy smell of vetiver makes a perfect signature scent for a man and imparts a sense of calm and focus.

Wisdom from the Garden

Vetiver oil comes from the roots of a grass native to India where it is known as the "oil of tranquility." Vetiver's long, tenacious root system contributes to its ability to combat erosion. Just as the plant itself is strong, the oil can strengthen and support us too. Vetiver helps create a focused environment and has been tested for its effectiveness on children with ADHD.[1] It can calm you when you need to sleep and free your mind from distraction when you need to concentrate.

Vetiver's smoky scent blends well with lavender, patchouli, clary sage, or ylang ylang in the diffuser.

Versatile, Viscous Vetiver

I often refer to diffusing as the gateway to oils for men. Many husbands in my oils group—my own included—love to use the diffuser. Bryan took one of ours to work a few months ago, and I know I'll never see it again unless I visit his office. My husband is one of those rare individuals who generally doesn't drink coffee, tea, or hot beverages, so his caffeine content is almost nonexistent. Diffusing at work helps wake him up, boost his immune system, or create a productive atmosphere—whichever he needs. As the plant manager of a manufacturing facility, his office sees a lot of traffic. He notices, however, that sometimes employees drop in just to stand over the diffuser.

Bryan fills our bedroom diffuser. Sometimes he gets in a rut, choosing the same oils night after night, and then he asks for suggestions. I frequently request vetiver combined with lavender or orange. Its smoky, relaxing aroma is calming and grounding. Roll-ons or diffuser blends created for focus often contain vetiver. As a lady in one of my oils groups described it, it's as if vetiver slows down the traffic in her mind.

Vetiver is thick. Carry the bottle in your bra or pocket for a few minutes before use to warm the oil, allowing it to drip easier. Add vetiver to your diffuser for a good night's sleep, blend with a carrier oil for a relaxing foot massage, or rub a drop on the back of your neck to calm down and relax.

Infused Living

Use vetiver to relax your mind and focus on the task at hand, whether it's studying for an exam, completing a difficult project, or blocking out distractions so you can hone in on the book you've finally made time to read.

ADD/ADHD AND FOCUS ROLLER

15 drops vetiver

15 drops lavender

15 drops cedarwood

Combine the oils in a 10-ml roller bottle and top it with coconut or other carrier oil. Roll on wrists, temples, back of the neck, or behind the ears for clarity, concentration, centering, or relief from test-taking jitters.

READING CORNER

3 drops vetiver

2 drops lavender

2 drops ylang ylang

FRESH RAIN

3 drops vetiver

6 drops lemon

> Add a few drops of vetiver oil to a warm bath to relax at bedtime.

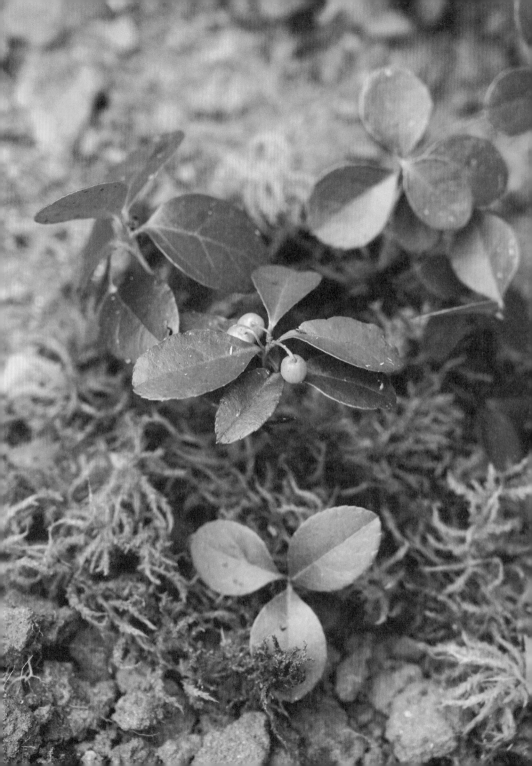

49

WINTERGREEN

The Essentials: *aromatic, topical, hot; avoid during pregnancy or for children under two*

Sweet, minty wintergreen possesses the wonderful combination of icy hotness that makes it perfect for pain relief. If you deal with physical discomfort, you may find wintergreen an effective, natural pain relief option.

Wisdom from the Garden

Wintergreen oil is steam distilled from the leaves and bark of the plant. North American Indians used wintergreen for colds, headaches, stomach aches, chronic indigestion, kidney disorders, and rheumatism. They made tea from the plant's leaves [1] and also chewed leaves for their flavor, to relieve aches and pains, and to increase respiratory capacity during hard work or when running long distances.[2] Wintergreen contains the powerful, naturally occurring chemical constituent methyl salicylate, which has analgesic and anti-inflammatory properties similar to aspirin. Wintergreen creates a cooling, soothing effect for topical pain relief and, when combined with peppermint oil, may be effective against low back pain.[3]

Wintergreen can be hot to the skin, so always combine it with a carrier oil. Because wintergreen is a highly concentrated plant extract with such an appealing scent, it should have a child-proof lid and be kept away from children. Companies seek to copy the benefits of methyl salicylate for commercial use by creating synthetic imitations for workout creams and to flavor gum and mints, but consumers beware. Avoid synthetics and use pure, therapeutic grade wintergreen essential oil.

The invigorating aroma of wintergreen blends well with basil, cypress, geranium, juniper, or peppermint in the diffuser.

Wonderful Wintergreen

One of the best things about my local oils group is the social aspect. We love to get together for classes, make-and-take parties, or oil-related DIYs. Anything to learn or talk about how to use our oils gives us an opportunity to hang out. Recently I hosted some diffuser bracelet workshops where we strung together lava rock beads and gemstones to make an assortment of beautiful custom jewelry. Once we finished tying together and gluing the ends, it was time to add essential oils to the lava rock beads. Because they are porous in nature, lava rock makes a perfect natural diffuser; adding oils to the beads enables you to smell the oil throughout the day. Put a drop or two of oil in your palm and roll the beads in it. This will cover more surface area and keep you from dripping it onto the string, which is more likely to break down with repeated exposure to oils.

A friend who was new to oils had a strong, almost physical reaction to two of the blends she inhaled. When I realized their common denominator was wintergreen, I fetched that bottle for her to smell too. Her reaction was equally strong. I've heard author Jen O'Sullivan say that a strong response to wintergreen can indicate the presence of pain. Your body craves the oil, a source of pain relief. When I asked my friend if she dealt with pain, she looked at me and with emphasis said, "Every day." She left my house with a new bracelet, an oils starter kit (I keep an extra on hand), and a plan to tackle her pain and out-of-whack hormones through natural means with oils, including wintergreen. I love researching, experimenting, and finding new solutions as old as the plants themselves, but it's a special thrill to help a friend discover them too. If you deal with physical pain, add wonderful wintergreen to your oils collection.

Infused Living

Add wintergreen to lotion or a carrier oil for a massage after working out. Apply it to your neck and shoulders or sore joints to invigorate you after an exhausting or stressful day.

CRAMPS BE GONE! PERIOD ROLLER

12 drops lavender
8 drops wintergreen
4 drops peppermint

Combine the oils in a 15-ml glass roller bottle and top with coconut or other carrier oil of your choice. Shake to combine. Roll on abdomen to relieve menstrual cramps.

SEA FOAM

3 drops lavender
3 drops rosemary
1 drop wintergreen

Diffuse the stimulating scent of wintergreen to clean and freshen the air.

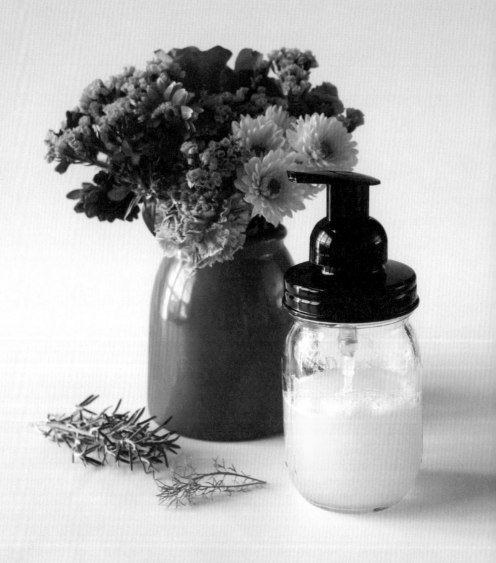

50

YLANG YLANG

The Essentials: *aromatic, topical*

When you add the sweet smell of ylang ylang to your health and beauty products, you can create a spa day at home. It's a signature scent that will make you feel beautiful!

Wisdom from the Garden

Not only is the pleasant and uplifting fragrance of ylang ylang—steam distilled from flowers of the tropical tree—used in many cosmetic products and perfumes, but it's also a natural aphrodisiac. In some cultures ylang ylang flowers, with their heady aroma, have been scattered over the bed of newlywed couples on their wedding night.

Ylang ylang has been shown to increase feelings of calmness, control blood pressure,[1] and lower stress, and it has been used for centuries as a natural hair thickener and to reduce hair loss.

Ylang ylang's rich, floral scent blends well with bergamot, orange, rosemary, cypress, or blue spruce in the diffuser.

Let him kiss me with the kisses of his mouth! For your love is better than wine;
your anointing oils are fragrant; your name is oil poured out.

Song of Solomon 1:2-3 ESV

The Desire of My Heart

I used to struggle with feelings of jealousy during weddings. I sat in the pew, tissue in hand, and imagined all the ways my own marriage might have started differently, better. I envied the bride who would return from her honeymoon and move into a house. We were married for 14 years before owning a home. I was jealous of the woman who entered marriage with financial security, which always eluded us. I allowed a day of happiness and celebration to stir embers of dissatisfaction within me.

You see, ours is a marriage of humble beginnings. We had a small wedding in my college town on a three-day weekend when Friday classes were canceled so that students could travel to an out-of-town football game. It required the full contents of my checking account to buy a dress off the rack and put Bryan's wedding ring on layaway.

Later we returned to our hometown in the months before and after our first child was born. Marriage and motherhood suited me, but I didn't realize how much my identity was tied up in being the smart, small-town girl who had ventured 1,800 miles from home to attend an Ivy League school. I was fulfilled yet humbled by my small, ordinary life.

Over the years I've continued to invest myself in both transitory and worldly identities—homeschooling mother of eight, Southerner, blogger—or worse, identities dependent on my skills or accomplishments: photographer, author, Russian major. First Peter 2:9 gives us both our identity—"a chosen generation, a royal priesthood, an holy nation, a peculiar people"—and our mission statement: "[to] shew forth the praises of him who hath called [us] out of darkness into his marvelous light." Our identity in Christ is the only one we can fully claim.

Keeping my priorities in order—God, husband, and then children and family—focuses the desires of my heart on both my Lord and my husband. Now I smile at weddings, through happy tears, and pray the new bride will be as blessed in her marriage as I am in mine.

Among the many blessings I enjoy, my husband refills our diffuser each night, usually with some mixture of lavender, cedarwood, and orange. But on those nights when I walk into an ylang ylang–infused room, it sends a signal to my brain, and I know it isn't sleep that's on his mind.

Infused Living

Do stress and schedules separate you and your husband? Plan a special time this week to show him he's still the desire of your heart. Dim the lights and diffuse ylang ylang to create a romantic atmosphere.

DIY FACE WASH

10 drops ylang ylang

5 drops rosemary

5 drops Roman chamomile

Ylang ylang is pronounced EE-lang EE-lang.

2/3 cup distilled water

1/3 cup Castile soap (coconut oil–free options are available, if you're allergic)

1 tsp. vitamin E oil

Combine the essential oils, Castile soap, and vitamin E oil in a foaming pump bottle and gently stir to combine. Top with distilled water, stir again, and top with a foaming soap pump.

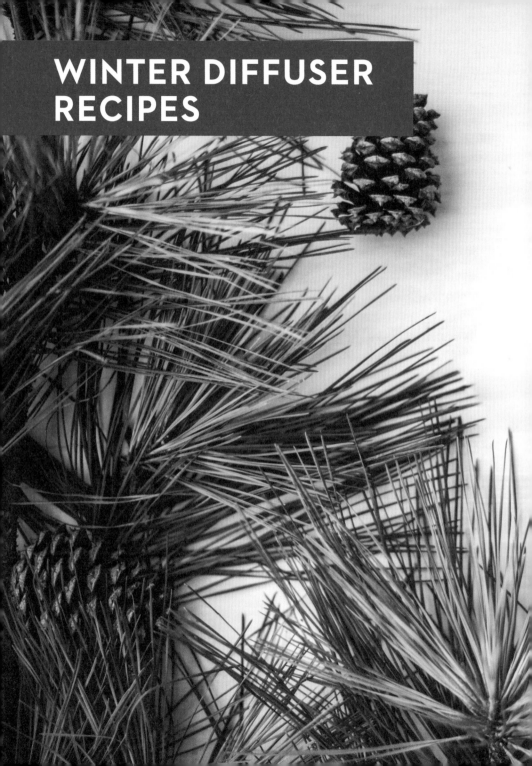

WINTER DIFFUSER RECIPES

WINTER FRESH

4 drops black spruce
4 drops orange
3 drops peppermint
2 drops clove

MULLED CIDER

4 drops orange
3 drops cinnamon bark
3 drops ginger

WINTER CHAI

3 drops orange
1 drop clove
1 drop nutmeg
1 drop cinnamon bark

SNOWFALL

4 drops wintergreen
2 drops pine
1 drop clove

WINTER WONDERLAND

2 drops frankincense
2 drops orange
2 drops juniper
2 drops grapefruit

LONG WINTER'S NAP

4 drops lavender
2 drops vetiver
2 drops cedarwood

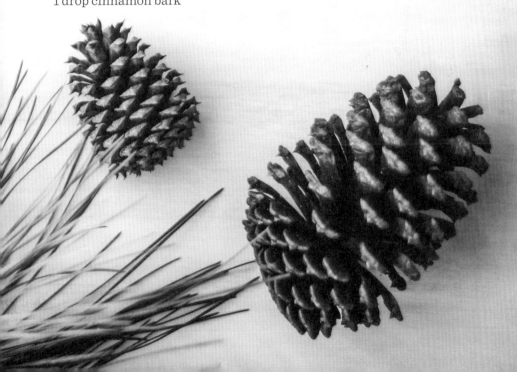

MY WISH FOR YOU

From the beginning, I've felt the Lord's leading in this project, and I hope my words have glorified Him and pointed you toward Him. I truly believe essential oils are God's gift to us.

I pray this book becomes a trusted reference in your home library and a roadmap on your path to natural health. If you want to delve into the world of oils but don't know where to start, I would love to share what my family uses. Contact me or visit itallbeganinagardenbook.com for more details. If this copy was given to you by a friend who uses oils, ask them questions about the quality standards of the company whose products they buy. Quality matters. We are unique individuals, and our bodies may respond differently to different oils, but to experience the benefits shown in this book, you need God's oils undiluted by man's synthetics.

Oil on, friend!
Dawn

Holy, holy, holy, is the Lord of hosts: the whole earth is full of his glory.

Isaiah 6:3

NOTES

How to Use This Book

[1] Stewart, David. *Healing Oils of the Bible* (Marble Hill, MO: The Center for Aromatherapy Research & Education, 2015), 16.

[2] Life Science Publishing, *Essential Oils Desk Reference, Seventh Edition* (Lehi, UT: Life Science Publishing, 2016), 17.

1. Basil

[1] Li, Hailong, et al. "Evaluation of the Chemical Composition, Antioxidant and Anti-Inflammatory Activities of Distillate and Residue Fractions of Sweet Basil Essential Oil." *Journal of Food Science and Technology*, Springer India, June 2017, www.ncbi.nlm.nih.gov/pubmed/28720944.

[2] Opalchenova, G., and D. Obreshkova. "Comparative Studies on the Activity of Basil—an Essential Oil from Ocimum Basilicum L.—against Multidrug Resistant Clinical Isolates of the Genera Staphylococcus, Enterococcus and Pseudomonas by Using Different Test Methods." *Journal of Microbiological Methods*, U.S. National Library of Medicine, July 2003, www.ncbi.nlm.nih.gov/pubmed/12732427.

[3] Satoh, Tomoko, and Yoshiaki Sugawara. "Effects on Humans Elicited by Inhaling the Fragrance of Essential Oils: Sensory Test, Multi-Channel Thermometric Study and Forehead Surface Potential Wave Measurement on Basil and Peppermint." *Analytical Sciences: The International Journal of the Japan Society for Analytical Chemistry*, U.S. National Library of Medicine, January 2003, www.ncbi.nlm.nih.gov/pubmed/12558038.

[4] Matiz, G., et al. "Effectiveness of Antimicrobial Formulations for Acne Based on Orange (Citrus Sinensis) and Sweet Basil (Ocimum Basilicum L) Essential Oils." *Biomedica: Revista Del Instituto Nacional De Salud*, U.S. National Library of Medicine, 2012, www.ncbi.nlm.nih.gov/pubmed/23235794.

[5] Gordon, Jerisha Parker. "Essential Oils for Menopause Relief: Does It Work?" *Healthline*, Healthline Media, 14 November 2018, www.healthline.com/health/menopause/essential-oils-for-menopause.

2. Bergamot

[1] Han, Xuesheng, et al. "Bergamot (Citrus Bergamia) Essential Oil Inhalation Improves Positive Feelings in the Waiting Room of a Mental Health Treatment Center: A Pilot Study." *Phytotherapy Research: PTR*, John Wiley and Sons Inc., May 2017, www.ncbi.nlm.nih.gov/pmc/articles/PMC5434918/.

[2] Levy, Jillian. "Stressed? Fatigued? Gaining Weight? You Might Have This Condition." *Dr. Axe*, 14 June 2018, draxe.com/cortisol-levels/.

3. Black Spruce

[1] Poaty, Bouddah, et al. "Composition, Antimicrobial and Antioxidant Activities of Seven Essential Oils from the North American Boreal Forest." *World Journal of Microbiology & Biotechnology*, U.S. National Library of Medicine, June 2015, www.ncbi.nlm.nih.gov/pubmed/25801172.

[2] Stewart, David. *Healing Oils of the Bible* (Marble Hill, MO: The Center for Aromatherapy Research & Education, 2015), 26-27.

[3] Levy, Jillian. "What Is the Limbic System? (Plus How to Keep It Healthy & the Role of Essential Oils)." *Dr. Axe*, 27 September 2016, draxe.com/health/brain-health/limbic-system/.

4. Blue Spruce

[1] Berardi, John, and Tom Nikkola. "What Do the Data Really Say about Essential Oils?" *Precision Nutrition*, 13 April 2018, www.precisionnutrition.com/what-do-the-data-really-say-about-essential-oils.

[2] Foust, Michael. "Boudia and Johnson Proclaim Christ on National TV after Winning Olympic Silver." *Christian Examiner Newspaper, Christian News, Christian Commentary, Church Events*, Christian Examiner, 8 August 2016, www.christianexaminer.com/article/boudia-and-johnson-proclaim-christ-on-national-tv-after-winning-silver/50949.htm.

5. Cedarwood

[1] Hartfield, Will. "The Truth About Using Cedar Wood Oil For Hair Loss." *Hair Loss Revolution*, 10 June 2019, www.hairlossrevolution.com/benefits-of-cedar-wood-oil-for-hair-growth/.

[2] Tobik, Amy K.D. "Best Essential Oils for Autism and ADHD—The Ultimate Guide." *Autism Parenting Magazine*, www.autismparentingmagazine.com/essential-oils-for-autism-adhd-add/.

6. Cinnamon Bark

[1] Urbaniak, A., et al. "The Antibacterial Activity of Cinnamon Oil on the Selected Gram-Positive and Gram-Negative Bacteria." *Current Neurology and Neuroscience Reports.*, U.S. National Library of Medicine, 2014, www.ncbi.nlm.nih.gov/pubmed/25369660.

[2] Johnson, Jon. "Essential Oils for Diabetes: Options and Aromatherapy." *Medical News Today*, MediLexicon International, 28 March 2019, www.medicalnewstoday.com/articles/317017.php.

7. Citronella

[1] De Toledo, Luciani Gaspar, et al. "Essential Oil of Cymbopogon Nardus (L.) Rendle: A Strategy to Combat Fungal Infections Caused by Candida Species." *International Journal of Molecular Sciences*, MDPI, 9 August 2016, www.ncbi.nlm.nih.gov/pubmed/27517903.

[2] Barhum, Lana. "Armpit Detox: Benefits and How to Do It." *Medical News Today*, MediLexicon International, 22 February 2018, www.medicalnewstoday.com/articles/319624.php.

[3] Heid, Markham. "5 Things Wrong With Your Deodorant." *Time*, Time, 5 July 2016, time.com/4394051/deodorant-antiperspirant-toxic/.

8. Clary Sage

[1] Deardeuff, LeAnne and David. *Taming the Dragon Within: How to Balance Women's Hormones with Essential Oils* (Lehi, UT: Life Science Publishing, 2014), 40.

[2] Deardeuff and Dearduff, *Taming the Dragon Within*, 30-33.

[3] Lee, Kyung-Bok, et al. "Changes in 5-Hydroxytryptamine and Cortisol Plasma Levels in Menopausal Women After Inhalation of Clary Sage Oil." *Phytotherapy Research: PTR*, U.S. National Library of Medicine, November 2014, www.ncbi.nlm.nih.gov/pubmed/24802524.

9. Clove

[1] "Eugenol." *National Center for Biotechnology Information, PubChem Compound Database*, U.S. National Library of Medicine, pubchem.ncbi.nlm.nih.gov/compound/Eugenol.

[2] Cai, L., and C.D. Wu. "Compounds from Syzygium Aromaticum Possessing Growth Inhibitory Activity against Oral Pathogens." *Journal of Natural Products*, U.S. National Library of Medicine, October 1996, www.ncbi.nlm.nih.gov/pubmed/8904847.

[3] Link, Rachael. "8 Surprising Health Benefits of Cloves." *Healthline*, Healthline Media, 26 August 2017, www.healthline.com/nutrition/benefits-of-cloves.

[4] Carlsen, Monica H, et al. "The Total Antioxidant Content of More than 3100 Foods, Beverages, Spices, Herbs and Supplements Used Worldwide." *Nutrition Journal*, BioMed Central, 22 January 2010, www.ncbi.nlm.nih.gov/pmc/articles/PMC2841576/.

[5] Stewart, David. *Healing Oils of the Bible* (Marble Hill, MO: The Center for Aromatherapy Research & Education, 2015), 17-18.

10. Copaiba

[1] Almeida, Mara Ribeiro, et al. "Genotoxicity Assessment of Copaiba Oil and Its Fractions in Swiss Mice." *Genetics and Molecular Biology*, Sociedade Brasileira De Genética, 2012, www.ncbi.nlm.nih.gov/pmc/articles/PMC3459418/.

[2] Guimarães, Anna Luísa Aguijar, et al. "Antimicrobial Activity of Copaiba (Copaifera Officinalis) and Pracaxi (Pentaclethra Macroloba) Oils against Staphylococcus Aureus: Importance in Compounding for Wound Care." *International Journal of Pharmaceutical Compounding*, U.S. National Library of Medicine, 2016, www.ncbi.nlm.nih.gov/pubmed/27125055.

[3] Gomes da Silva, Ary, et al. "Application of the Essential Oil from Copaiba (Copaifera Langsdori Desf.) for Acne Vulgaris: A Double-Blind, Placebo-Controlled Clinical Trial." *Alternative Medicine Review: A Journal of Clinical Therapeutic*, U.S. National Library of Medicine, March 2012, www.ncbi.nlm.nih.gov/pubmed/22502624.

[4] Souza, Ariana B., et al. "Antimicrobial Evaluation of Diterpenes from Copaifera Langsdorffii Oleoresin Against Periodontal Anaerobic Bacteria." *Molecules* (Basel, Switzerland), MDPI, 18 November 2011, www.ncbi.nlm.nih.gov/pmc/articles/PMC6264602/.

11. Cypress

[1] Boukhris, Maher, et al. *Chemical Composition and Biological Potential of Essential Oil from Tunisian Cupressus Sempervirens*, L. 2012, nodaiweb.university.jp/desert/pdf/JALS-P74_329-332.pdf.

[2] Ahmed Ali, Sanaa, et al. "Protective Role of Juniperus Phoenicea and Cupressus Sempervirens Against CCl(4)." *World Journal of Gastrointestinal Pharmacology and Therapeutics*, Baishideng Publishing Group Co., Limited, 6 December 2010, www.ncbi.nlm.nih.gov/pubmed/21577307.

[3] Ferguson, Sian. "All About Cypress Oil: Science, Benefits, Risks & How to Use It." *Healthline*, Healthline Media, 17 April 2019, www.healthline.com/health/cypress-oil.

[4] Butnariu, Monica, and Ioan Sarac. "Essential Oils From Plants." *Journal of Biotechnology and Biomedical Science*, Open Access Pub, 21 December 2018, openaccesspub.org/jbbs/article/940.

[5] O'Sullivan, Jen. *The Essential Oil Truth: The Facts Without the Hype* (Jen O'Sullivan/31 Oils, LLC, 2018) 15.

12. Davana

[1] "Scent of Danger: Are There Toxic Ingredients in Perfumes and Colognes?" *Scientific American*, 29 September 2012, www.scientificamerican.com/article/toxic-perfumes-and-colognes/.

[2] Sifferlin, Alexandra. "Phthalates Linked to Lower Thyroid Function in Girls: Study." *Time*, Time, 31 May 2017, time.com/4799330/household-chemicals-phthalates-thyroid-girls/.

[3] "Should People Be Concerned about Parabens in Beauty Products?" *Scientific American*, 6 October 2014, www.scientificamerican.com/article/should-people-be-concerned-about-parabens-in-beauty-products/.

[4] "5 Things to Know About Triclosan." *U.S. Food and Drug Administration*, FDA, www.fda.gov/consumers/consumer-updates/5-things-know-about-triclosan.

[5] "Talcum Powder and Cancer." *American Cancer Society*, www.cancer.org/cancer/cancer-causes/talcum-powder-and-cancer.html.

13. Elemi

[1] Mogana, R., and C. Wiart. "Canarium L.: A Phytochemical and Pharmacological Review." *Journal of Pharmacy Research*, June 2011, jprsolutions.info/files/final-file-57a09ac95944b3.23842686.pdf.

14. Eucalyptus

[1] Pletcher, Peggy. "9 Amazing Eucalyptus Oil Benefits You Need to Know." *Healthline*, Healthline Media, 25 July 2017, www.healthline.com/health/9-ways-eucalyptus-oil-can-help.

[2] Saporito, F., et al. "Essential Oil-Loaded Lipid Nanoparticles for Wound Healing." *International Journal of Nanomedicine*, 2018, www.ncbi.nlm.nih.gov/pubmed/29343956.

15. Fennel

[1] Alexandrovich, Irina, et al. "The Effect of Fennel (Foeniculum Vulgare) Seed Oil Emulsion in Infantile Colic: A Randomized, Placebo-Controlled Study." *Alternative Therapies in Health and Medicine*, U.S. National Library of Medicine, 2003, www.ncbi.nlm.nih.gov/pubmed/12868253.

[2] Liu, Qing, et al. "Antibacterial and Antifungal Activities of Spices." *International Journal of Molecular Sciences*, MDPI, 16 June 2017, www.ncbi.nlm.nih.gov/pmc/articles/PMC5486105/.

[3] Group, Edward. "The Weight Loss Benefits of Fennel Seed Essential Oil." *Dr. Group's Healthy Living Articles*, 14 October 2015, www.globalhealingcenter.com/natural-health/weight-loss-benefits-fennel-seed-essential-oil/.

[4] Harvard Health Publishing. "Can Gut Bacteria Improve Your Health?" *Harvard Health*, October 2016, www.health.harvard.edu/staying-healthy/can-gut-bacteria-improve-your-health.

17. Geranium

[1] Orchard, Ané, and Sandy van Vuuren. "Commercial Essential Oils as Potential Antimicrobials to Treat Skin Diseases." *Evidence-Based Complementary and Alternative Medicine: ECAM*, Hindawi, 2017, www.ncbi.nlm.nih.gov/pmc/articles/PMC5435909/.

[2] Shinohara, Kazuyuki, et al. "Effects of Essential Oil Exposure on Salivary Estrogen Concentration in Perimenopausal Women." *Neuro Endocrinology Letters*, U.S. National Library of Medicine, January 2017, www.ncbi.nlm.nih.gov/pubmed/28326753.

[3] Lotfipur Rafsanjani, Seyede Maryam, et al. "Comparison of the Efficacy of Massage and Aromatherapy Massage with Geranium on Depression in Postmenopausal Women: A Clinical Trial." *Zahedan Journal of Research in Medical Sciences*. April 2015, https://pdfs.semanticscholar.org/7d67/420308e57a936c7cfd64a44f022f8152f82b.pdf.

18. Ginger

[1] Lua, Pei Lin, et al. "Effects of Inhaled Ginger Aromatherapy on Chemotherapy-Induced Nausea and Vomiting and Health-Related Quality of Life in Women with Breast Cancer." *Complementary Therapies in Medicine*, U.S. National Library of Medicine, June 2015, www.ncbi.nlm.nih.gov/pubmed/26051575.

[2] Townsend, Elizabeth A, et al. "Effects of Ginger and Its Constituents on Airway Smooth Muscle Relaxation and Calcium Regulation." *American Journal of Respiratory Cell and Molecular Biology*, American Thoracic Society, February 2013, www.ncbi.nlm.nih.gov/pmc/articles/PMC3604064/.

[3] Sritoomma, Netchanok, et al. "The Effectiveness of Swedish Massage with Aromatic Ginger Oil in Treating Chronic Low Back Pain in Older Adults: A Randomized Controlled Trial." *Complementary Therapies in Medicine*, U.S. National Library of Medicine, February 2014, www.ncbi.nlm.nih.gov/pubmed/24559813.

[4] Mashhadi, Nafiseh Shokri, et al. "Anti-Oxidative and Anti-Inflammatory Effects of Ginger in Health and Physical Activity: Review of Current Evidence." *International Journal of Preventive Medicine*, Medknow Publications & Media Pvt Ltd, April 2013, www.ncbi.nlm.nih.gov/pmc/articles/PMC3665023/.

19. Grapefruit

[1] "The 5 Best Essential Oils for Weight Loss." *U.S. News & World Report*, U.S. News & World Report, 2 May 2017, health.usnews.com/health-news/blogs/eat-run/articles/2017-05-02/the-5-best-essential-oils-for-weight-loss.

[2] Uysal, Burcu, et al. "Essential Oil Composition and Antibacterial Activity of the Grapefruit (Citrus Paradisi. L) Peel Essential Oils Obtained by Solvent-Free Microwave Extraction: Comparison with Hydrodistillation." *International Journal of Food Science & Technology*, John Wiley & Sons, Ltd (10.1111), 27 April 2011, onlinelibrary.wiley.com/doi/abs/10.1111/j.1365-2621.2011.02640.x.

[3] Niijima, Akira, and Katsuya Nagai. "Effect of Olfactory Stimulation with Flavor of Grapefruit Oil and Lemon Oil on the Activity of Sympathetic Branch in the White Adipose Tissue of the Epididymis." *Experimental Biology and Medicine* (Maywood, N.J.), U.S. National Library of Medicine, November 2003, www.ncbi.nlm.nih.gov/pubmed/14610259.

[4] O'Sullivan, Jen. *The Essential Oil Truth: The Facts Without the Hype* (Jen O'Sullivan/31 Oils, LLC, 2018), 28.

[5] Stiles, K.G. *The Essential Oils Complete Reference Guide: Over 250 Recipes for Natural Wholesome Aromatherapy* (Salem, MA: Page Street Publishing Co., 2017), 222.

20. Helichrysum

[1] Orchard, Ané, and Sandy van Vuuren. "Commercial Essential Oils as Potential Antimicrobials to Treat Skin Diseases." *Evidence-Based Complementary and Alternative Medicine: ECAM*, Hindawi, 2017, www.ncbi.nlm.nih.gov/pmc/articles/PMC5435909/.

[2] Lorenzi, Vannina, et al. "Geraniol Restores Antibiotic Activities against Multidrug-Resistant Isolates from Gram-Negative Species." *Antimicrobial Agents and Chemotherapy*, American Society for Microbiology Journals, 1 May 2009, aac.asm.org/content/53/5/2209.long.

[3] Lourens, A.C.U., et al. "In Vitro Biological Activity and Essential Oil Composition of Four Indigenous South African Helichrysum Species." *Journal of Ethnopharmacology*, U.S. National Library of Medicine, December 2004, www.ncbi.nlm.nih.gov/pubmed/15507345.

[4] "16 of the Absolute Best Essential Oils for Headaches." *Pain Doctor*, 1 June 2017, paindoctor.com/essential-oils-for-headaches/.

21. Hyssop

[1] Fathiazad, Fatemeh, et al. "Phytochemical Analysis and Antioxidant Activity of Hyssopus Officinalis L. from Iran." *Advanced Pharmaceutical Bulletin*, Tabriz University of Medical Sciences, 2011, www.ncbi.nlm.nih.gov/pubmed/24312758.

[2] Stanković, Nemanja, et al. "Comparative Study of Composition, Antioxidant, and Antimicrobial Activities of Essential Oils of Selected Aromatic Plants from Balkan Peninsula." *Planta Medica*, U.S. National Library of Medicine, May 2016, www.ncbi.nlm.nih.gov/pubmed/26891001.

[3] Stewart, David. *Healing Oils of the Bible* (Marble Hill, MO: The Center for Aromatherapy Research & Education, 2015), 292-293.

22. Jasmine

[1] Hongratanaworakit, Tapanee. "Stimulating Effect of Aromatherapy Massage with Jasmine Oil." *Natural Product Communications*, U.S. National Library of Medicine, January 2010, www.ncbi.nlm.nih.gov/pubmed/20184043.

[2] "Smell of Jasmine 'as Calming as Valium'." *The Telegraph*, Telegraph Media Group, 10 July 2010, www.telegraph.co.uk/news/science/7881819/Smell-of-jasmine-as-calming-as-valium.html.

[3] Orchard, Ané, and Sandy van Vuuren. "Commercial Essential Oils as Potential Antimicrobials to Treat Skin Diseases." *Evidence-Based Complementary and Alternative Medicine: ECAM*, Hindawi, 2017, www.ncbi.nlm.nih.gov/pmc/articles/PMC5435909/.

23. Juniper

[1] "Juniper." *Gale Encyclopedia of Alternative Medicine*, Encyclopedia.com, 2019, www.encyclopedia.com/plants-and-animals/plants/plants/juniper.

[2] Keville, Kathy. "Aromatherapy: Juniper Berry." *HowStuffWorks*, HowStuffWorks, 30 April 2007, health.howstuffworks.com/wellness/natural-medicine/aromatherapy/aromatherapy-juniper-berry.htm.

[3] Shenefelt, Philip D. "Herbal Treatment for Dermatologic Disorders." *Herbal Medicine: Biomolecular and Clinical Aspects. 2nd Edition.*, U.S. National Library of Medicine, 1 January 1970, www.ncbi.nlm.nih.gov/books/NBK92761/.

[4] White, Adrian. "Essential Oil for Burns: Lavender, Peppermint, Best, and More." *Healthline*, Healthline Media, 1 November 2018, www.healthline.com/health/essential-oil-for-burns#best-essential-oils.

[5] Cronkleton, Emily. "Try 18 Essential Oils for Sore Muscles." *Healthline*, Healthline Media, 15 May 2019, www.healthline.com/health/fitness-exercise/essential-oils-for-sore-muscles.

[6] Purdie, Jennifer. "Can You Use Essential Oils for Weight Loss?" *Healthline*, Healthline Media, 27 July 2017, www.healthline.com/health/diet-and-weight-loss/essential-oils-for-weight-loss.

[7] "Juniper." *Gale Encyclopedia of Alternative Medicine*, Encyclopedia.com, 2019, www.encyclopedia.com/plants-and-animals/plants/plants/juniper.

24. Lavender

[1] Phung, Alice Chi. "René-Maurice Gattefossé Archives." *D-Brief*, 10 February 2015, blogs
.discovermagazine.com/scienceandfood/2015/02/10/lavender/.

[2] Kianpour, M., et al. "Effect of Lavender Scent Inhalation on Prevention of Stress, Anxiety and Depression in
the Postpartum Period." *Iran J Nurs Midwifery Res*, 2016, https://www.ncbi.nlm.nih.gov/pmc/articles/
PMC4815377/.

25. Lemon

[1] Komiya, Migiwa, et al. "Lemon Oil Vapor Causes an Anti-Stress Effect via Modulating the 5-HT and DA
Activities in Mice." *Behavioural Brain Research*, U.S. National Library of Medicine, 25 September 2006,
www.ncbi.nlm.nih.gov/pubmed/16780969.

26. Lemongrass

[1] Boukhatem, Mohamed Nadjib, et al. "Lemon Grass (Cymbopogon Citratus) Essential Oil as a Potent
Anti-Inflammatory and Antifungal Drugs." *The Libyan Journal of Medicine*, Co-Action Publishing, 19
September 2014, www.ncbi.nlm.nih.gov/pmc/articles/PMC4170112/.

[2] Agbafor, K.N., & Akubugwo, E.I. "Hypocholesterolaemic Effect of Ethanolic Extract of Fresh Leaves of
Cymbopogon Citratus (Lemongrass)." *African Journal of Biotechnology*, Academic Journals, 5 March
2007, academicjournals.org/journal/AJB/article-abstract/6AE822C6504.

[3] Zouhir, Abdelmajid, et al. "Inhibition of Methicillin-Resistant Staphylococcus Aureus (MRSA) by
Antimicrobial Peptides (AMPs) and Plant Essential Oils." *Pharmaceutical Biology*, U.S. National
Library of Medicine, December 2016, www.ncbi.nlm.nih.gov/pubmed/27246787.

[4] O'Sullivan, Jen. *Vitality: The Young Living Lifestyle* (Scotts Valley, CA: CreateSpace, 2018), 52.

27. Lime

[1] Preedy, Victor R., ed., *Essential Oils in Food Preservation, Flavor and Safety* (Cambridge, MA: Academic
Press, 2016), 531-537.

[2] Amorim, Jorge Luis, et al. "Anti-Inflammatory Properties and Chemical Characterization of the Essential
Oils of Four Citrus Species." *PloS One*, Public Library of Science, 18 Apr. 2016, www.ncbi.nlm.nih.gov/
pubmed/27088973.

28. Manuka

[1] Orchard, A., et al. "The in Vitro Antimicrobial Evaluation of Commercially Essential Oils and Their
Combinations against Acne." *International Journal of Cosmetic Science*, U.S. National Library of
Medicine, 24 March 2018, www.ncbi.nlm.nih.gov/pubmed/29574906.

[2] Turchi, Barbara, et al. "Sub-Inhibitory Stress with Essential Oil Affects Enterotoxins Production and
Essential Oil Susceptibility in Staphylococcus Aureus." *Natural Product Research*, U.S. National
Library of Medicine, March 2018, www.ncbi.nlm.nih.gov/pubmed/28595460.

[3] Chen, Chien-Chia, et al. "Investigations of Kanuka and Manuka Essential Oils for *in Vitro* Treatment of
Disease and Cellular Inflammation Caused by Infectious Microorganisms." *Journal of Microbiology,
Immunology and Infection*, Elsevier, 28 February 2014, www.sciencedirect.com/science/article/pii/
S1684118213002466.

[4] Krader, Kate. "A Cult New Zealand Honey Is Causing Legal Problems in the U.S." *Bloomberg .com*, Bloomberg, 26 August 2018, www.bloomberg.com/news/articles/2018-08-26/ the-new-zealand-honey-that-s-causing-legal-problems-in-the-u-s.

29. Myrrh

[1] Stewart, David. *Healing Oils of the Bible* (Marble Hill, MO: The Center for Aromatherapy Research & Education, 2007), 139.

[2] Freeman, Jennifer. "RA Essential Oils: What Essential Oils Are Anti-Inflammatory?" *RheumatoidArthritis.org*, 27 October 2018, www.rheumatoidarthritis.org/living-with-ra/diet/ essential-oils/.

[3] Gadir, Suad A., and Ibtisam M. Ahmed. "Commiphora Myrrha and Commiphora Africana Essential Oils." *Journal of Chemical and Pharmaceutical Research*, 2014, www.jocpr.com/articles/commiphora-myrrha-and-commiphora-africana-essential-oils.pdf.

[4] Haffor, Al-Said A. "Effect of Commiphora Molmol on Leukocytes Proliferation in Relation to Histological Alterations before and during Healing from Injury." *Saudi Journal of Biological Sciences*, U.S. National Library of Medicine, April 2010, www.ncbi.nlm.nih.gov/pubmed/23961070.

[5] Feng, Jie, et al. "Identification of Essential Oils with Strong Activity against Stationary Phase *Borrelia Burgdorferi.*" *Antibiotics* (Basel, Switzerland), MDPI, 16 October 2018, www.ncbi.nlm.nih.gov/ pubmed/30332754.

30. Myrtle

[1] Alipour, Ghazal, et al. "Review of Pharmacological Effects of Myrtus Communis L. and Its Active Constituents." *Phytotherapy Research*, vol. 28, no. 8, 2014, pp. 1125-1136., doi:10.1002/ptr.5122.

[2] Stewart, David. *The Chemistry of Essential Oils Made Simple* (Marble Hill, MO: Care Publications, 2013), 60.

31. Nutmeg

[1] Abourashed, Ehab A., and Abir T El-Alfy. "Chemical Diversity and Pharmacological Significance of the Secondary Metabolites of Nutmeg (*Myristica Fragrans* Houtt.)." *Phytochemistry Reviews: Proceedings of the Phytochemical Society of Europe*, U.S. National Library of Medicine, December 2016, www.ncbi .nlm.nih.gov/pmc/articles/PMC5222521/.

[2] Zhang, Chuan-Rui, et al. "Antioxidant and Antiinflammatory Compounds in Nutmeg (Myristicafragrans) Pericarp as Determined by in Vitro Assays." *Natural Product Communications*, U.S. National Library of Medicine, August 2015, www.ncbi.nlm.nih.gov/pubmed/26434127.

[3] Shafiei, Zaleha, et al. "Antibacterial Activity of Myristica Fragrans against Oral Pathogens." *Evidence-Based Complementary and Alternative Medicine: ECAM*, Hindawi, 2012, www.ncbi.nlm.nih.gov/pmc/ articles/PMC3434417/.

[4] Kubala, Jillian. "8 Science-Backed Benefits of Nutmeg." *Healthline*, Healthline Media, 12 June 2019, www .healthline.com/nutrition/nutmeg-benefits.

[5] Naidoo, Uma. "Spice up Your Holidays with Brain-Healthy Seasonings." *Harvard Health Blog*, 22 November 2016, www.health.harvard.edu/blog/spice-up-your-holidays-with-brain-healthy-seasonings-2016120710734.

33. Oregano

[1] Béjaoui, Afef, et al. "Essential Oil Composition and Antibacterial Activity of Origanum Vulgare Subsp. Glandulosum Desf. at Different Phenological Stages." *Journal of Medicinal Food*, Mary Ann Liebert, Inc., December 2013, www.ncbi.nlm.nih.gov/pmc/articles/PMC3868303/.

[2] De Castro, Ricardo Dias, et al. "Antifungal Activity and Mode of Action of Thymol and Its Synergism with Nystatin Against Candida Species Involved with Infections in the Oral Cavity: An in Vitro Study." *BMC Complementary and Alternative Medicine*, BioMed Central, 24 November 2015, bmccomplementalternmed.biomedcentral.com/articles/10.1186/s12906-015-0947-2.

[3] Nordqvist, Joseph. "Oregano: Health Benefits, Uses, and Side Effects." *Medical News Today*, MediLexicon International, 11 December 2017, www.medicalnewstoday.com/articles/266259.php.

34. Palmarosa

[1] Janbaz, K.H., et al. "Bronchodilator, Vasodilator and Spasmolytic Activities of Cymbopogon Martinii." *Journal of Physiology and Pharmacology: An Official Journal of the Polish Physiological Society*, U.S. National Library of Medicine, December 2014, www.ncbi.nlm.nih.gov/pubmed/25554990.

[2] Pérez-Rosés, Renato, et al. "Biological and Nonbiological Antioxidant Activity of Some Essential Oils." *Journal of Agricultural and Food Chemistry*, U.S. National Library of Medicine, 15 June 2016, www.ncbi.nlm.nih.gov/pubmed/27214068.

[3] Andrade, Murbach Teles, et al. "Cymbopogon Martinii Essential Oil and Geraniol at Noncytotoxic Concentrations Exerted Immunomodulatory/Anti-Inflammatory Effects in Human Monocytes." *The Journal of Pharmacy and Pharmacology*, U.S. National Library of Medicine, October 2014, www.ncbi.nlm.nih.gov/pubmed/24934659.

[4] Gemeda, Negero, et al. "Development, Characterization, and Evaluation of Novel Broad-Spectrum Antimicrobial Topical Formulations from *Cymbopogon Martini* (Roxb.) W. Watson Essential Oil." *Evidence-Based Complementary and Alternative Medicine: ECAM*, Hindawi, 10 September 2018, www.ncbi.nlm.nih.gov/pubmed/30275867.

[5] Stewart, David. *Healing Oils of the Bible* (Marble Hill, MO: The Center for Aromatherapy Research & Education, 2015), 27-28.

[6] Ansari, M.A., and R.K. Razdan. "Relative Efficacy of Various Oils in Repelling Mosquitoes." *Indian Journal of Malariology*, U.S. National Library of Medicine, September 1995, www.ncbi.nlm.nih.gov/pubmed/8936292.

[7] O'Sullivan, Jen. *The Essential Oil Truth: The Facts Without the Hype* (Jen O'Sullivan/31 Oils, LLC, 2018), 21.

36. Peppermint

[1] Meamarbashi, Abbas, and Ali Rajabi. "The Effects of Peppermint on Exercise Performance." *Journal of the International Society of Sports Nutrition*, BioMed Central, 21 March 2013, www.ncbi.nlm.nih.gov/pmc/articles/PMC3607906/.

[2] Moss, Mark, et al. "Modulation of Cognitive Performance and Mood by Aromas of Peppermint and Ylang-Ylang." *Intern. J. Neuroscience*, 2008, www.dr-hatfield.com/educ538/docs/moss+2008.pdf.

37. Pine

[1] Zeng, Wei-Cai, et al. "Chemical Composition, Antioxidant, and Antimicrobial Activities of Essential Oil from Pine Needle (Cedrus Deodara)." *Journal of Food Science*, U.S. National Library of Medicine, July 2012, www.ncbi.nlm.nih.gov/pubmed/22757704.

[2] Mühlbauer, R.C., et al. "Common Herbs, Essential Oils, and Monoterpenes Potently Modulate Bone Metabolism." *Bone*, U.S. National Library of Medicine, April 2003, www.ncbi.nlm.nih.gov/pubmed/12689680.

[3] "Cleaning Supplies and Household Chemicals." *American Lung Association*, www.lung.org/our-initiatives/healthy-air/indoor/indoor-air-pollutants/cleaning-supplies-household-chem.html.

[4] Steinemann, A.C., et al., "Fragranced Consumer Products: Chemicals Emitted, Ingredients Unlisted." *Environmental Impact Assessment Review*, 2010, journalistsresource.org/wp-content/uploads/2011/10/Steinemann-et-al.-2010.pdf.

38. Roman Chamomile

[1] Sándor, Zsolt, et al. "Evidence Supports Tradition: The *in Vitro* Effects of Roman Chamomile on Smooth Muscles." *Frontiers in Pharmacology*, Frontiers Media S.A., 6 April 2018, www.ncbi.nlm.nih.gov/pubmed/29681854.

[2] Patzelt-Wenczler, R., and E. Ponce-Pöschl. "Proof of Efficacy of Kamillosan(R) Cream in Atopic Eczema." *European Journal of Medical Research*, U.S. National Library of Medicine, 19 April 2000, www.ncbi.nlm.nih.gov/pubmed/10799352.

[3] Piccaglia, Roberta, et al. "Antibacterial and Antioxidant Properties of Mediterranean Aromatic Plants." *Industrial Crops and Products*, Elsevier, 23 September 2003, www.sciencedirect.com/science/article/abs/pii/0926669093900107.

[4] Saderi, Horieh, et al. "Antimicrobial Effects of Chamomile Extract and Essential Oil on Clinically Isolated Porphyromonas gingivalis from Periodontitis." Acta Hort, 2004, volume 6, https://www.actahort.org/books/680/680_21.htm.

[5] Zhao, Jianping, et al. "Octulosonic Acid Derivatives from Roman Chamomile (Chamaemelum Nobile) with Activities against Inflammation and Metabolic Disorder." *Journal of Natural Products*, U.S. National Library of Medicine, 28 March 2014, www.ncbi.nlm.nih.gov/pubmed/24471493.

[6] "Roman Chamomile: Uses, Side Effects, Dosage, Interactions & Health Benefits." *EMedicineHealth*, www.emedicinehealth.com/roman_chamomile/vitamins-supplements.htm.

[7] Wilkinson, S., et al. "An Evaluation of Aromatherapy Massage in Palliative Care." *Palliative Medicine*, U.S. National Library of Medicine, September 1999, www.ncbi.nlm.nih.gov/pubmed/10659113.

[8] Kong, Yingying, et al. "Inhalation of Roman Chamomile Essential Oil Attenuates Depressive-like Behaviors in Wistar Kyoto Rats." *Science China, Series C Life Sciences*, U.S. National Library of Medicine, June 2017, www.ncbi.nlm.nih.gov/pubmed/28527112.

39. Rose

[1] Hongratanaworakit, Tapanee. "Relaxing Effect of Rose Oil on Humans." *Natural Product Communications*, U.S. National Library of Medicine, February 2009, www.ncbi.nlm.nih.gov/pubmed/19370942.

[2] Orchard, Ané, and Sandy van Vuuren. "Commercial Essential Oils as Potential Antimicrobials to Treat Skin Diseases." *Evidence-Based Complementary and Alternative Medicine: ECAM*, Hindawi, 2017, www.ncbi.nlm.nih.gov/pmc/articles/PMC5435909/.

[3] Stewart, David. *Healing Oils of the Bible* (Marble Hill, MO: The Center for Aromatherapy Research & Education, 2007), 31-32.

[4] O'Sullivan, Jen. *The Essential Oil Truth: The Facts Without the Hype* (Jen O'Sullivan/31 Oils, LLC, 2018), 28-30.

[5] If you like, you can purchase *Essential of Parfumerie* at https://melissapoepping.com/shop-1/essential-parfumerie.

41. Sage

[1] "Sage Benefits & Information (Salvia Officinalis)." *Herbwisdom*, www.herbwisdom.com/herb-sage.html.

[2] Bommer, S., et al. "First Time Proof of Sage's Tolerability and Efficacy in Menopausal Women with Hot Flushes." *SpringerLink*, Springer Healthcare Communications, 16 May 2011, link.springer.com/article/10.1007%2Fs12325-011-0027-z.

42. Sandalwood

[1] Kyle, Gaye. "Evaluating the Effectiveness of Aromatherapy in Reducing Levels of Anxiety in Palliative Care Patients: Results of a Pilot Study." *Complementary Therapies in Clinical Practice*, U.S. National Library of Medicine, May 2006, www.ncbi.nlm.nih.gov/pubmed/16648093.

[2] "Sandalwood Scent Facilitates Wound Healing and Skin Regeneration." *EurekAlert!*, 8 July 2014, www.eurekalert.org/pub_releases/2014-07/rb-ssf070814.php.

[3] Warnke, Patrick H., et al. "The Battle against Multi-Resistant Strains: Renaissance of Antimicrobial Essential Oils as a Promising Force to Fight Hospital-Acquired Infections." *Journal of Cranio-Maxillofacial Surgery*, volume 37, issue 7, October 2009, www.sciencedirect.com/science/article/abs/pii/S1010518209000523.

[4] Moy, Ronald L., and Corey Levenson. "Sandalwood Album Oil as a Botanical Therapeutic in Dermatology." *The Journal of Clinical and Aesthetic Dermatology*, Matrix Medical Communications, October 2017, www.ncbi.nlm.nih.gov/pmc/articles/PMC5749697/.

[5] Stewart, David. *Healing Oils of the Bible* (Marble Hill, MO: The Center for Aromatherapy Research & Education, 2015), 140.

[6] Stewart, David. *Healing Oils of the Bible*, 73.

43. Spearmint

[1] O'Sullivan, Jen. *Vitality: The Young Living Lifestyle* (Scotts Valley, CA: CreateSpace, 2018), 46.

44. Tangerine

[1] Lv, Xinmiao, et al. "Citrus Fruits as a Treasure Trove of Active Natural Metabolites That Potentially Provide Benefits for Human Health." *Chemistry Central Journal*, Springer International Publishing, 24 December 2015, www.ncbi.nlm.nih.gov/pmc/articles/PMC4690266/.

45. Tea Tree

[1] Orchard, Ané, and Sandy van Vuuren. "Commercial Essential Oils as Potential Antimicrobials to Treat Skin Diseases." *Evidence-Based Complementary and Alternative Medicine: ECAM*, Hindawi, 2017, www.ncbi.nlm.nih.gov/pmc/articles/PMC5435909/.

[2] Kamath, N.P., et al. "The Effect of Aloe Vera and Tea Tree Oil Mouthwashes on the Oral Health of School Children." *European Archives of Paediatric Dentistry: Official Journal of the European Academy of Paediatric Dentistry*, U.S. National Library of Medicine, 20 May 2019, www.ncbi.nlm.nih.gov/pubmed/31111439.

[3] "The Hidden Health Hazards of Plug-In Air Fresheners." *IndoorDoctor*, 21 March 2017, www.indoordoctor.com/health-hazards-plug-air-fresheners/.

46. Thyme

[1] Langeveld, W.T., et al. "Synergy Between Essential Oil Components and Antibiotics: A Review." *Critical Reviews in Microbiology*, February 2014, https://www.ncbi.nlm.nih.gov/pubmed/23445470.

47. Valerian

[1] Cropley, M., et al. "Effect of Kava and Valerian on Human Physiological and Psychological Responses to Mental Stress Assessed under Laboratory Conditions." *Phytotherapy Research: PTR*, U.S. National Library of Medicine, February 2002, www.ncbi.nlm.nih.gov/pubmed/11807960.

[2] Taavoni, S., et al. "Valerian/Lemon Balm Use for Sleep Disorders during Menopause." *Complementary Therapies in Clinical Practice*, U.S. National Library of Medicine, November 2013, www.ncbi.nlm.nih.gov/pubmed/24199972.

[3] Mirabi, Parvaneh, and Faraz Mojab. "The Effects of Valerian Root on Hot Flashes in Menopausal Women." *Iranian Journal of Pharmaceutical Research: IJPR*, Shaheed Beheshti University of Medical Sciences, 2013, www.ncbi.nlm.nih.gov/pubmed/24250592.

[4] Moghadam, Zahra Behboodi, et al. "The Effect of Valerian Root Extract on the Severity of Pre Menstrual Syndrome Symptoms." *Journal of Traditional and Complementary Medicine*, Elsevier, 19 January 2016, www.ncbi.nlm.nih.gov/pubmed/27419099.

48. Vetiver

[1] Friedmann, Terry S. *Attention Deficit and Hyperactivity Disorder (ADHD)*. 2002, files.meetup.com/1481956/ADHD%20Research%20by%20Dr.%20Terry%20Friedmann.pdf.

49. Wintergreen

[1] "Wildflowers of the Adirondacks: Wintergreen (Gaultheria Procumbens)." *Adirondack Wildflowers: Wintergreen (Gaultheria Procumbens)*, wildadirondacks.org/adirondack-wildflowers-wintergreen-gaultheria-procumbens.html.

[2] *Healthy Ingredients: Wintergreen*, American Botanical Council, cms.herbalgram.org/healthyingredients/Wintergreen.html.

[3] Hebert, Patricia R., et al. "Treatment of Low Back Pain: the Potential Clinical and Public Health Benefits of Topical Herbal Remedies." *Journal of Alternative and Complementary Medicine (New York, N.Y.)*, Mary Ann Liebert, Inc., 1 April 2014, www.ncbi.nlm.nih.gov/pmc/articles/PMC3995208/.

50. Ylang Ylang

[1] Jung, Da-Jung, et al. "Effects of Ylang-Ylang Aroma on Blood Pressure and Heart Rate in Healthy Men." *Journal of Exercise Rehabilitation*, 25 April 2013, https://www.ncbi.nlm.nih.gov/pmc/articles/PMC3836517/.